VEGETARIAN COOKBOOK

VEGETARIAN RECIPES THAT ARE HEALTHY AND EASY TO MAKE

DIANA POLSKA

CONTENTS

Tasty Potato and Pancetta Breakfast 11
Special Breakfast Omelet 13
Berry Smoothie 15
Breakfast Smoothie 17
Breakfast Fruits Salad 19
Tomato and Feta Omelet 21
Elegant Vegetarian Breakfast 23
Orange Salad 25
Green Tofu Scramble 27
Breakfast Salad with Tahini and Lime 29
Grapefruit Salad 31
Salmon and Broccoli Frittata 33
Fruit Compote 35
Easy Breakfast Ratatouille 37
Coconut Granola 39
Delicious Chia Pudding 41
Spinach and Quinoa Muffins 43
Breakfast Bowl 45
Special Cranberry Nut Bread 47
Incredible Poppy Scones 49
Tasty Breakfast Potatoes 51
Breakfast Oatmeal 53
Breakfast Tomato and Basil Quiche 55
Breakfast Pumpkin Smoothie 57
Carrot Muffins 59
Tasty Aubergine and Pepper Pilaf 61
Tasty Green Soup 63
Delicious Cabbage and Fennel Seed Mix 65
Chili Bean Soup 67
Indian Potato Dish 69
Special Barley Risotto 71
Stuffed Squash 73
Halloumi Salad 75
Amazing Sweet Potatoes with Chickpeas Dish 77
Delicious Poached Potatoes 79
Vegetable Dish 81
Asparagus and Potato Frittata 83
Special Surprise Dish 85
Asparagus and Courgette Salad 87
Tasty Pepper and Bean Salad 89
Tasty Potato Soup 91
Easy Vegetable Dish 93

Mushroom Gratin....95
Tasty Tuscan Soup....97
Eggs and Chips....99
Spicy Butternut Soup....101
Mushroom Pilaf....103
Potato Tortilla....105
Delicious Potatoes and Black Beans....107
Beetroot Salad....109
Kale Salad....111
Delightful Stuffed Marrow....113
Stuffed Peppers....115
Bean Tostadas....117
Tomato Soup....119
Mushroom and Greens Stew....121
Healthy Bean Soup....123
Tasty Lunch Cucumber Salad....125
Delicious Lettuce and Fennel Salad....127
Tasty Barley Soup....129
Carrot and Coriander Soup....131
Turkish Style Vegetarian Salad....135
Tofu and Eggplant Packages....137
Avocado and Goat Cheese Quesadilla....139
Amazing Mexican Rice....141
Vegetarian Chili with Peppers....143
Vegetarian Burritos....145
Vegetarian Salad Boats....147
Mexican Style Quinoa Burgers....149
Gourmet Porridge with Cilantro....151
Lunch Omelet Wrap....153
Gourmet Lunch Salad....155
Grain Salad with Avocado Dressing....157
Beans, Caramelized Onions, and Almonds....159
Delicious Tomato and Peach Salad....161
Wow Salad....163
Fancy Zucchini Dish....165
Artichoke Pizza....167
Tofu Sandwiches....169
Cucumber and Watermelon Salad....171
Fresh Tomato Salad....173
Okra and Potato Dish....175
Indian Style Okra....177
Grilled Squash with Delicious Salsa....179
Dinner Salad with Tasty Garlic Dressing....181
Avocado Salad....183
Dinner Vegetarian Curry....185

Dinner Tofu Stew.......187
Thai Vegan Pumpkin Stew.......189
Broccoli and Quinoa Dish.......191
Delicate Dinner Salad.......193
Vegetarian Pad Thai.......195
Vegetarian Dinner Gazpacho.......197
Dinner Pea Salad.......199
Special Dinner Pasta.......201
Fennel and Apple Salad.......203
Tasty Roasted Celery.......205
Roasted Spring Onions.......207
Delicious Mashed Potatoes.......209
Amazing Potato Salad.......211
Grilled Vegetables with Special Glaze.......213
Vegetable Croquettes.......215
Delicious Farfalle with Tomatoes.......217
Vegetarian Stuffed Potatoes.......219
Dinner Mix.......221
Potato Pancakes.......223
Barley Salad.......225
Greens with Artichoke Vinaigrette.......227
Delightful Dinner.......229
Vegetable Sheppard's Pie.......231
Spinach and Ricotta Gnocchi.......233
Wonderful Bread Salad.......235
Tomato Burger.......237
Vegetable Noodles and Tasty Coconut Sauce.......239
Asparagus and Special Mushroom Mayonnaise.......241
Cauliflower Dhal.......243
Stir Fry Cabbage Mix.......245
Chunky Vegetable Salad.......247
Special Cauliflower and Chickpea Curry.......249
Ricotta with Pomodoro Sauce.......251
Chickpea Tagine and Figs.......253
Caramelized Onion Tart.......255
Special Vegetable Pies.......257
Vegetarian Maple Cupcakes.......259
Baked Apples.......261
Pumpkin Cookies.......263
Tasty Curd.......265
Delicious Rhubarb Pie.......267
Cherry Cobbler.......269
Fruit Salad.......271
Fruit Jelly.......273
Couscous Dessert.......275

Fruit Cocktail 277
Fig and Almond Dessert..279
Avocado Dessert Salad 281
Vegetarian Sponge Cake 283
Pumpkin Pie 285
Apple and Pumpkin Dessert..287
Blueberry and Coconut Cake..289
Baked Nectarine and Almond Dessert..291
Vegetarian Passion Fruit Pudding 293
Cornbread Muffins 295
Fruits with Orange Vinaigrette..297
Delicious Cherry Sorbet 299
Vegetarian Apricot Sorbet 301
Mango Granita 303
Apple Crisp 305
Grapefruit Granita 307

RECIPES

Tasty Potato and Pancetta Breakfast

Potatoes and pancetta are the best combinations ever!

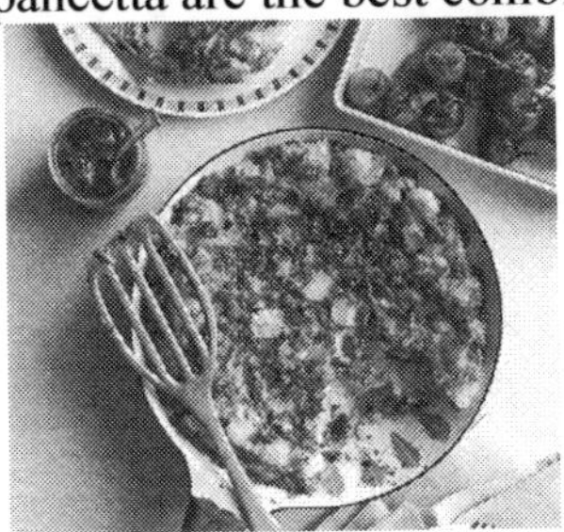

Ingredients:
28 ounces of gold potatoes, cut into large chunks
Water for boiling
1 yellow onion, finely chopped
1½ tablespoon of extra-virgin olive oil
2 garlic cloves, finely chopped
3 ounces of pancetta, finely diced
2 ounces of gruyere, finely grated
2 eggs, whisked
Salt and black pepper to taste
A small bunch of parsley, finely chopped
Some cherry tomatoes, already roasted for serving

Directions:

1. Put potatoes in a pot. Cover with water. Add salt. Put heat on medium-high. Simmer for 15 minutes.
2. Heat up ½ tablespoons of olive oil in a pot, over low heat. Cook onion and garlic for 15 minutes. Stir constantly.
3. Remove onion and garlic from pan. Add pancetta. Cook for 3-4 minutes.
4. Drain potatoes. Chop them into small cubes and put them in a bowl.
5. Add sautéed onion and garlic, pancetta, gruyere, eggs, salt, pepper, and parsley. Stir well.
6. Heat up a pan with the rest of the oil. Add potato mix. Cook at a low temperature for 15 minutes.
7. Flip. Cook for 15 more minutes.
8. Transfer food to a plate. Serve with roasted tomatoes.

Enjoy!

Nutritional value: 350 calories, 15 grams of fat, 30 grams of carbs, 10 grams of protein, 4 grams of fiber

Special Breakfast Omelet

It's the best vegetarian breakfast ever!

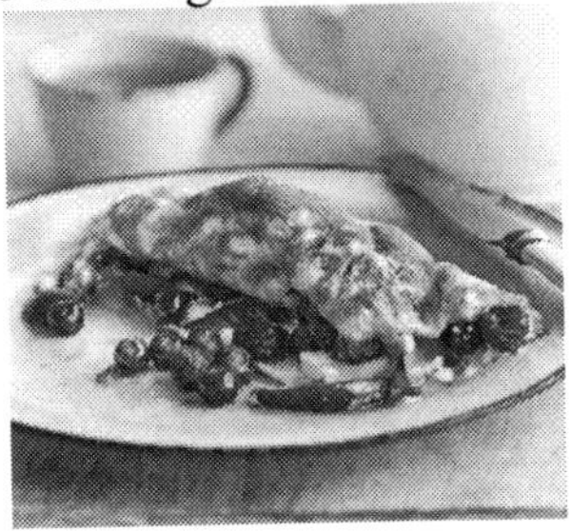

Ingredients:
1 egg
½ teaspoon of rapeseed oil
3 pinches of cinnamon
1 tablespoon of almond milk
3 ounces of cottage cheese
4 ounces of mixed strawberries, raspberries, and blueberries

Directions:

1. In a bowl, whisk the egg with milk and cinnamon.
2. Heat up a pan at a medium-high temperature. Add egg mix. Swirl to cover pan. Cook for 2 minutes. Transfer to a plate.
3. Spread cheese and berries over omelet. Roll. Serve right away.

Enjoy!

Nutritional value: 200 calories, 10 grams of fat, 4 grams of fiber, 20 grams of protein, 18 grams of carbs

Berry Smoothie

It's the best way to start your day!

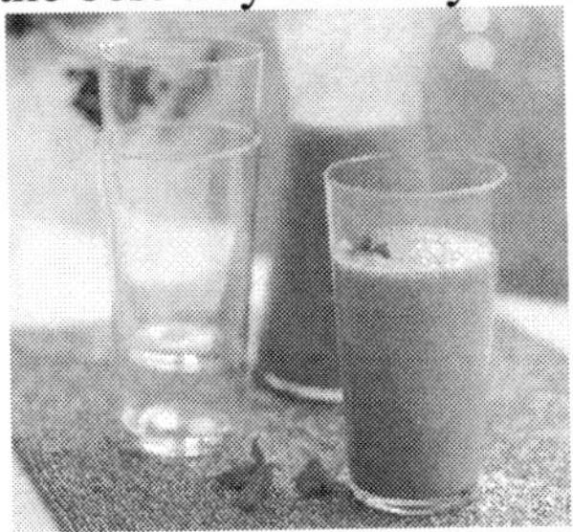

Ingredients:
7 ounces of cranberry juice
6 ounces of raspberries
3 ounces of almond milk
6 ounces of natural yogurt
1 tablespoon of palm sugar
Some mint sprigs for serving

Directions:

1. Put the raspberries in your blender.
2. Add cranberry juice, milk, yogurt and sugar. Pulse well.
3. Pour into a glass. Serve with mint springs.

Enjoy!

Nutritional value: 100 calories, 2 grams of fat, 1 grams of fiber, 5 grams of protein, 16 grams of carbs

Breakfast Smoothie

Try a new day with a new and tasty smoothie!

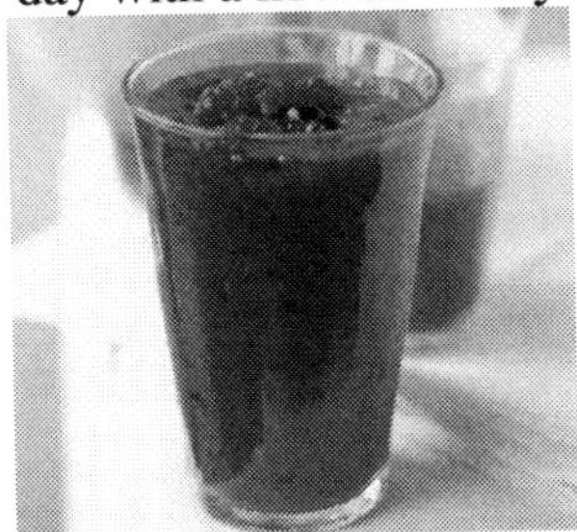

Ingredients:
1 large banana, sliced
5 ounces of blackberries
A splash of mineral water
Runny honey for serving

Directions:

1. Put the banana in your blender. Pulse a few times.
2. Add blackberries. Mix again.
3. Add mineral water. Pulse for 10 seconds. Transfer to a tall glass. Serve with honey on top.

Enjoy!

Nutritional value: 123 calories, 0 grams of fat, 28 grams of carbs, 3 grams of fiber, 2 grams of protein

Breakfast Fruits Salad

This salad is easy to make and it's so healthy!

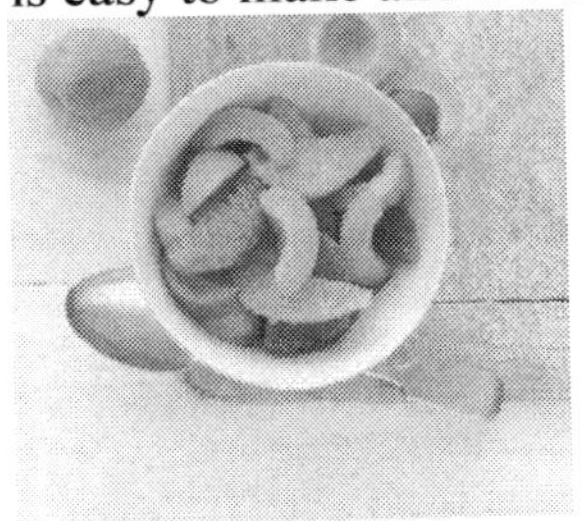

Ingredients:
4 oranges, sliced
2 grapefruits, sliced
4 apricots, sliced
1 tablespoon of honey

Directions:

1. Put oranges in a salad bowl.
2. Add grapefruits and apricots.
3. Drizzle honey on top. Toss to coat.
4. Serve right away!

Enjoy!

Nutritional value: 83 calories, 0 grams of fat, 18 grams of carbs, 4 grams of fibers, 2 grams of protein

Tomato and Feta Omelet

It's a quick breakfast that will give you enough energy to face a busy day!

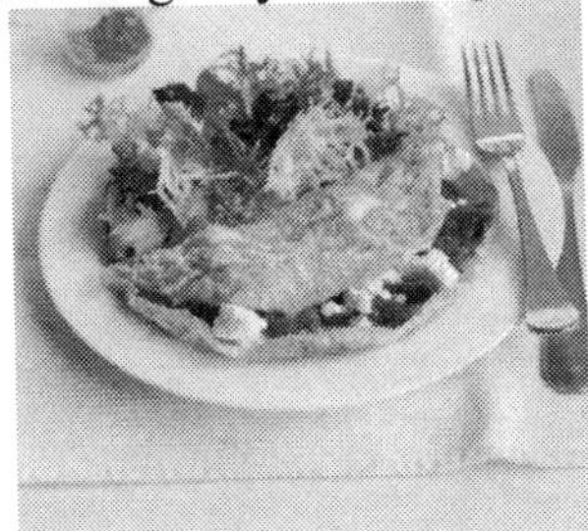

Ingredients:
4 sun-dried tomatoes, chopped
2 eggs, whisked
1 teaspoon of extra-virgin olive oil
A small handful of mixed salad leaves
½ tablespoon of feta cheese, crumbled

Directions:

1. Heat up a pan with olive oil at a medium-high temperature. Add eggs. Scramble them.
2. Add tomatoes and feta cheese. Stir again.
3. Cook for 1 more minute. Transfer to a plate. Serve with mixed salad leaves.

Enjoy!

Nutritional value: 240 calories, 20 grams of fat, 5 grams of carbs, 1 gram of fibers, 18 grams of protein

Elegant Vegetarian Breakfast

It's such a rich meal! What are you waiting for? Try it now!

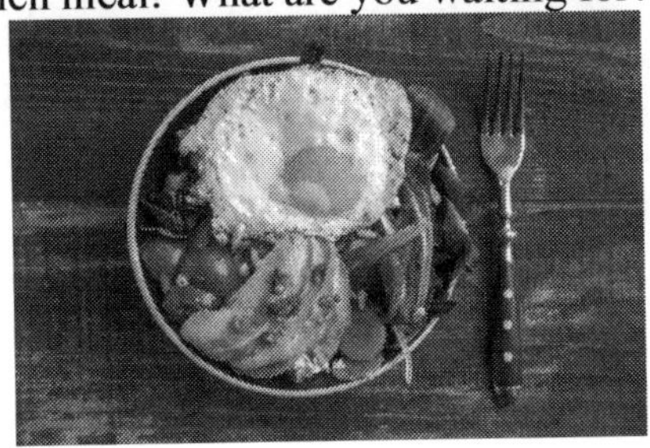

Ingredients:
2 handfuls of cherry tomatoes, halved
1 medium cucumber, thickly sliced
1 avocado, diced
1 red bell pepper, chopped
1 sprigs basil, roughly chopped
1 sprigs parsley, chopped
1 tablespoon of extra-virgin olive oil
¼ cup of pine nuts, toasted
Sea salt to taste
2 eggs
Some vegetable oil for frying

Directions:

1. In a salad bowl, mix cucumber with tomatoes, bell pepper, avocado, basil, parsley, and nuts. Stir gently.
2. Add olive oil and salt to taste. Toss to coat.
3. Meanwhile, heat up a pan with some vegetable oil at a medium-high temperature. Crack eggs. Fry them.
4. Transfer eggs on top of salad. Serve right away!

Enjoy!

Nutritional value: 240 calories, 38 grams of fat, 30 grams of carbs, 13 grams of fibers, 15 grams of protein

Orange Salad

It's a fresh and healthy breakfast!

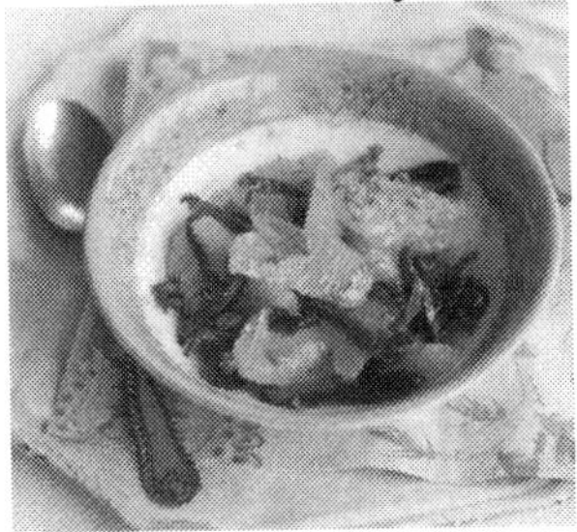

Ingredients:
12 dates, cut lengthwise
4 oranges, sliced
A small bunch of mint, finely chopped
1 tablespoon of rosewater

Directions:

1. Put oranges and dates in a salad bowl.
2. Add mint and rosewater. Toss to coat.
3. Serve right away with some mint leaves on top.

Enjoy!

Nutritional value: 120 calories, 1 grams of fat, 50 grams of carbs, 5 grams of fibers, 4 grams of protein

Green Tofu Scramble

This mix will become your new favorite breakfast!

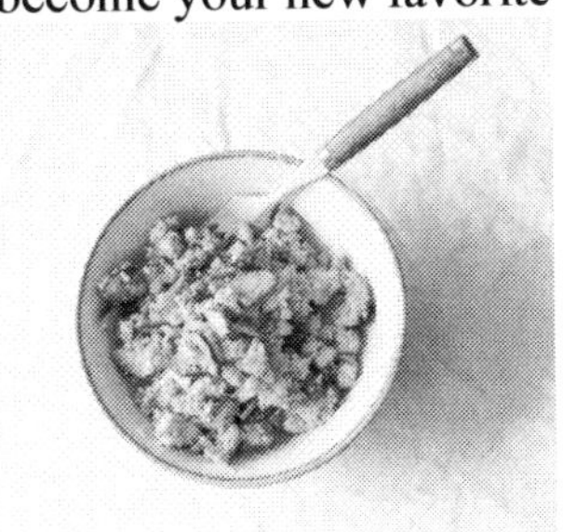

Ingredients:
1 cup of yellow onion, chopped
1 tablespoon of extra-virgin olive oil
1 cup of zucchini, chopped
16 ounces of firm tofu, pressed and crumbled
10 ounces of spinach, chopped
2 tablespoons of tahini paste
3 tablespoons of nutritional yeast
½ teaspoon of turmeric
Sea salt and black pepper to taste
3 tablespoons of water

Directions:

1. Heat up a pan with the oil at a medium-high temperature. Cook onion for 2-3 minutes.
2. Add zucchini. Stir and cook for 5 more minutes.
3. Add tofu and spinach. Stir and cook for 1 minute.
4. Add tahini, yeast, turmeric, salt, pepper and 3 tablespoons of water.
5. Stir. Keep on the stove for 1-2 minutes more. Transfer to serving plates. Serve!

Enjoy!

Nutritional value: 144 calories, 5 grams of fat, 11 grams of carbs, 3 grams of fiber, 1 grams of protein

Breakfast Salad with Tahini and Lime

It's a delicious salad suitable for a busy person!

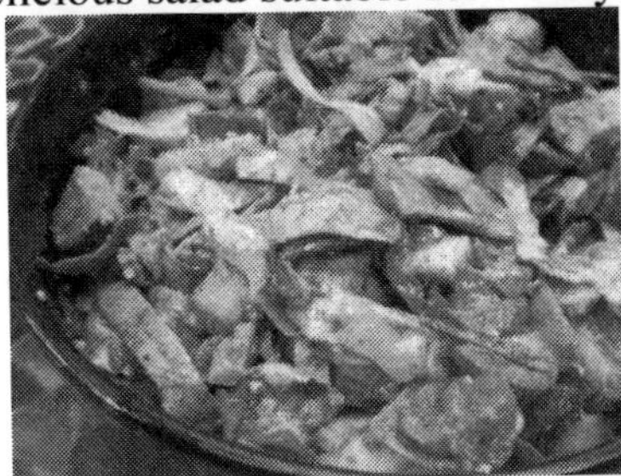

Ingredients:
5 lettuce leaves, roughly chopped
1 peach, chopped
1 cup of baby spinach, chopped
½ mango, chopped
10 strawberries, cut in halves
1 tablespoon of hemp seeds
1 cucumber, sliced
For the dressing:
1 tablespoon of lime juice
1 tablespoon of tahini
1 tablespoon of date syrup
1 tablespoon of coconut water
½ teaspoon of spirulina powder

Directions:

1. In a salad bowl, mix lettuce leaves with spinach, mango, peach, cucumber, strawberries and hemp seeds.
2. In a small bowl, mix lime juice with date syrup, tahini, coconut water and spirulina powder. Stir well.
3. Add dressing to the salad. Toss to coat. Serve right away!

Enjoy!

Nutritional value: 130 calories, 2 grams of fat, 3 grams of fiber, 3 grams of protein

Grapefruit Salad

Few ingredients. Simple recipe.

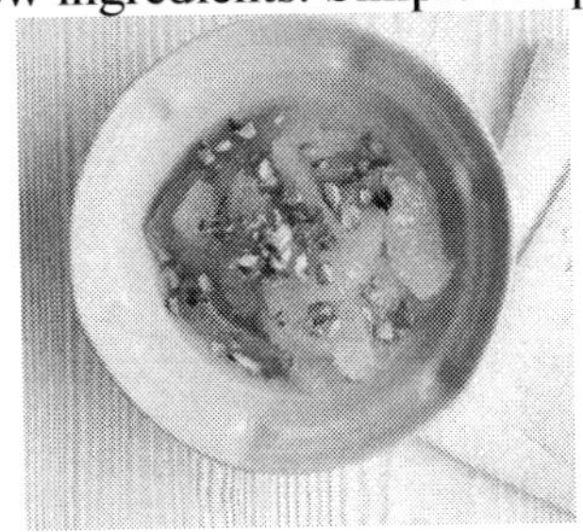

Ingredients:
1 white grapefruit, sliced
1 pink grapefruit, sliced
1 teaspoon of pistachios, chopped
1 tablespoon of agave nectar

Directions:

1. Put grapefruit slices in a salad bowl.
2. Add pistachio and agave nectar. Toss to coat. Serve right away!

Enjoy!

Nutritional value: 107 calories, 1 grams of fat, 21 grams of carbs, 2 grams of fibers, grams of proteins 2

Salmon and Broccoli Frittata

It's an elegant and filling recipe! You need to make it right now!

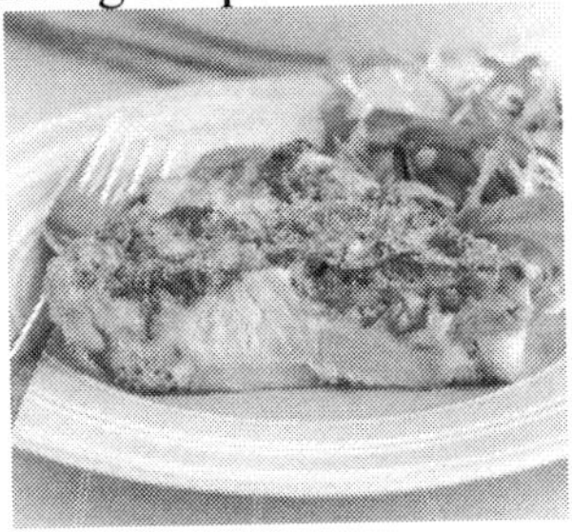

Ingredients:
17 ounces of potatoes, roughly chopped
1 tablespoon of olive oil
2 skinless salmon fillets
1 small head broccoli, cut into florets
8 eggs, whisked
A small handful of mint, finely chopped

Directions:

1. Put potatoes in a pot. Cover with water. Place on the stove at a medium-high temperature. Boil for 12 minutes.
2. After 8 of the 12 minutes have passed, add the broccoli.
3. Drain potatoes and broccoli when they are tender enough. Transfer to a bowl. Leave aside.
4. Place salmon fillets in an oven proof dish. Put them in the microwave for 3 minutes.
5. Heat up a pan with the oil at a medium-high temperature. Add chopped potatoes. Cook for 3 minutes.
6. Flake salmon. Add to potatoes. Stir well.
7. Add broccoli, mint, salt, pepper and eggs.
8. Stir well. Cook for 6 minutes. Transfer to a plate. Serve right away!

Nutritional value: 340 calories, 20 grams of fat, 20 grams of carbs, 34 grams of protein

Fruit Compote

It's time for something really tasty: a breakfast fruit compote.

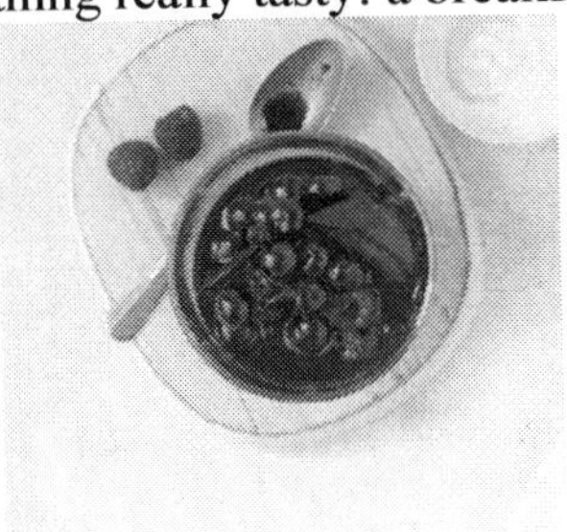

Ingredients:
Zest from 1 lemon
Juice from 1 lemon
4 large plums, cut in wedges
7 ounces of punnet blueberry
5 ounces of punnet raspberry
½ tablespoon of palm sugar
4 tablespoons of water

Directions:

1. Put plums and blueberries in a pan. Heat up at a medium temperature. Mix with lemon juice and zest. Cook for 4 minutes.
2. Add the water, sugar and the raspberries. Cook for 1 more minute.
3. Take compote off heat. Allow it to cool down. Serve with a drizzle of honey.

Enjoy!

Nutritional value: 98 calories, 22 grams of carbs, 4 grams of fiber, 2 grams of protein

Easy Breakfast Ratatouille

It's such a hearty meal that you won't need to eat anything else for the rest of the day!

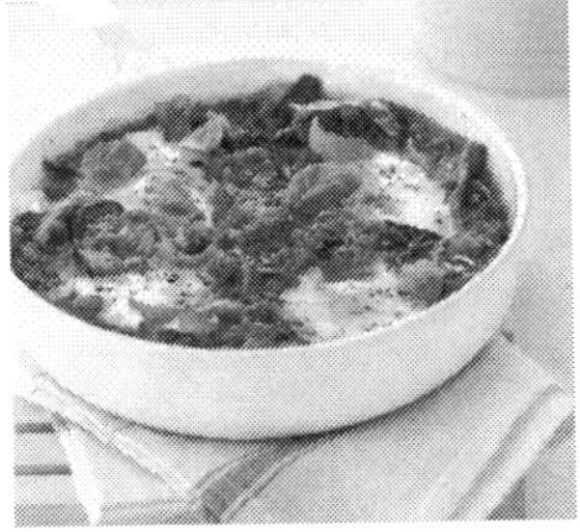

Ingredients:
1 yellow onion, chopped
1 tablespoon of extra-virgin olive oil
1 red bell pepper, sliced
2 garlic cloves, finely chopped
1 aubergine, chopped
1 tablespoon of rosemary, finely chopped
2 courgettes, chopped
1 teaspoon of balsamic vinegar
A sprigs basil, roughly chopped
4 eggs
Salt and black pepper to taste
14 ounces of diced canned tomatoes

Directions:

1. Heat up a pan with the oil at a medium-high temperature. Cook pepper, garlic, onion, rosemary for 5 minutes. Stir constantly.
2. Add courgettes and aubergine. Cook for 2 more minutes.
3. Add tomatoes. Bring to a boil. Cover. Simmer for 20 minutes, then uncover and simmer for 20 minutes more.
4. Add vinegar and eggs. Season with salt and pepper. Cover pot. Cook for 5 minutes.
5. Sprinkle basil on top. Serve right away!

Enjoy!

Nutritional value: 190 calories, 11 grams of fat, 13 grams of carbs, 5 grams of fibers, 12 grams of protein

Coconut Granola

It's such an easy recipe! You'll love it!

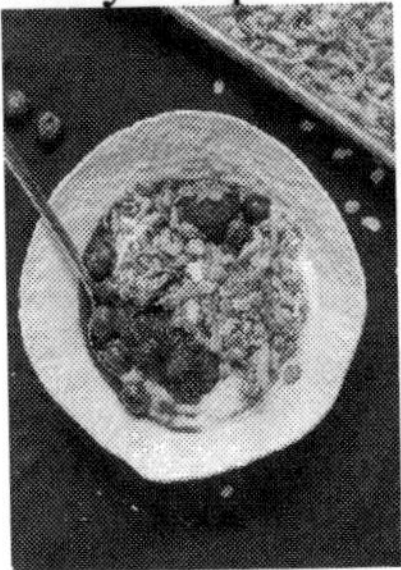

Ingredients:
4 cups of rolled oats
1 teaspoon of cinnamon
1 cup of almonds
½ teaspoon of ground ginger
¾ teaspoon of sea salt
½ cup of coconut oil
½ cup of maple syrup
1 teaspoon of vanilla extract
½ cup of unsweetened coconut flakes
½ cup of unsweetened, shredded coconut

Directions:

1. In a bowl, mix oats with salt, ginger, almonds and cinnamon. Stir well.
2. Add coconut oil, vanilla, and maple syrup. Stir well.
3. Transfer this mix to a baking sheet lined with parchment paper. Spread evenly.
4. Put food in the oven at 350 degrees F. Bake for 15 minutes.
5. Remove from the oven. Add coconut and coconut flakes. Stir everything.
6. Put food in the oven. Bake for 5 more minutes.
7. Take granola out of the oven. Leave it to cool down. Serve.

Enjoy!

Nutritional value: 81 calories, 4 grams of fat, 9 grams of carbs, 1 grams of fiber, 1 grams of protein

Delicious Chia Pudding

It's a creamy and healthy pudding! Try it for breakfast tomorrow!

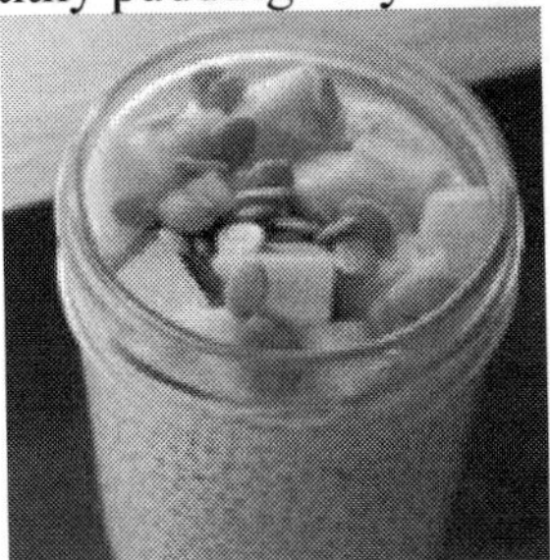

Ingredients:
¼ cup of chia seeds
6 dates
1½ cups of water
2/3 cup of cashews, soaked in water for 2 hours and drained
A pinch of sea salt
½ teaspoon of cinnamon
½ teaspoon of vanilla extract
Sliced fruits for serving

Directions:

1. In a bowl, mix chia seeds with water. Cover. Leave aside for 15 minutes.
2. In a blender, mix dates with cinnamon, salt, cashews and vanilla. Pulse a few times.
3. Pour half of the chia. Pulse some more.
4. Transfer into serving bowls. Top with the rest of the chia seeds. Garnish with your favorite fruits.

Enjoy!

Nutritional value: 120 calories, 7 grams of fat, 10 grams of carbs, 6 grams of protein

Spinach and Quinoa Muffins

The combination is just perfect! You won't regret it!

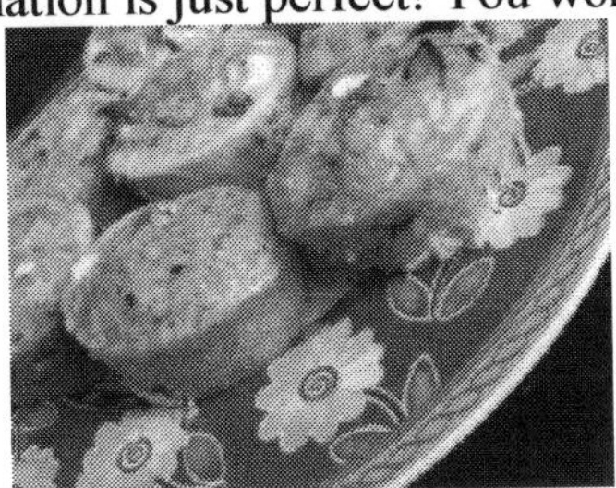

Ingredients:
1 cup of quinoa
2 cups of water
1 cup of spinach
1 small yellow onion, chopped
2 eggs
¼ cup of grated cheese
½ teaspoon of garlic powder
Sea salt and black pepper to taste
½ teaspoon of oregano
Cooking spray

Directions:

1. Put water in a saucepan. Heat it up. Add quinoa. Cover. Bring to a boil. Simmer for 10 minutes.
2. Remove from heat. Leave aside for now.
3. Heat up a pan at a medium-high temperature. Add onion. Cook for 2-3 minutes.
4. Add spinach. Cook for 2 more minutes. Take off heat. Leave aside.
5. In a bowl, mix quinoa with spinach and onion mixture, eggs, cheese, salt, pepper, garlic powder, and oregano. Stir well.
6. Grease a muffin pan with some cooking spray. Pour mixture into it. Put food in the oven at 350 degrees F. Bake for 20 minutes.
7. Take muffins out of the oven. Leave aside to cool down. Then serve!

Enjoy!

Nutritional value: 9 calories, 2 grams of fats, 1 gram of carbs, 1 grams of fiber, 4 grams of protein

Breakfast Bowl

Start your day with a super breakfast!

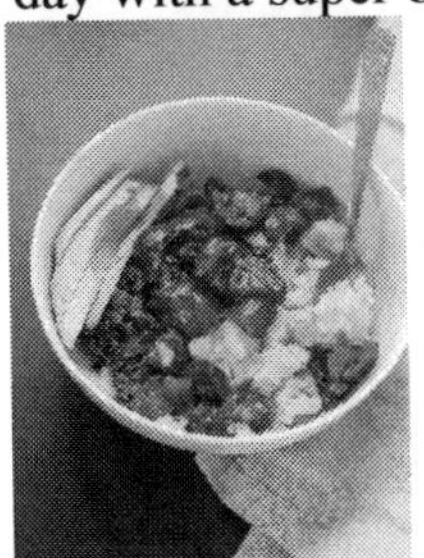

Ingredients:

For pico de gallo:

1 pint of cherry tomatoes, cut in quarters
¼ cup of chopped cilantro
¼ cup of white onion, finely chopped
A pinch of sea salt
1 tablespoon of lime juice

For the refried black beans:

½ cup of white onion, finely chopped
1 tablespoon of olive oil
2 teaspoons of cumin
30 ounces of canned black beans, drained
2 garlic cloves, finely chopped
½ cup of water
1 teaspoon of lime juice
Salt and black pepper to taste

For the eggs:

10 eggs
Salt and black pepper to taste
A pinch of red pepper flakes
2 teaspoons of olive oil
Your favorite salsa for serving

Directions:

1. In a bowl, mix tomatoes with a ¼ cup of white onion, chopped cilantro, a pinch of sea salt and 1 tablespoon of lime juice. Stir well. Leave aside.
2. Heat up a pan with 1 tablespoon of olive oil at a medium-high temperature. Cook ½ cup of white onion for 7-8 minutes. Stir constantly.
3. Add cumin, garlic and a pinch of salt. Stir well.
4. After 1 minute, add beans and water. Stir. Cover. Cook for 5 more minutes.
5. Reduce heat. Mash half of the beans using a fork. Cook for 3 minutes.
6. Remove from heat. Season with salt and pepper. Add 1 teaspoon of lime juice. Stir. Leave aside.
7. Meanwhile, in a bowl, mix eggs with salt, pepper, and red pepper flakes.

8. Heat up a pan with 2 teaspoons of olive oil. Add egg mixture to pan. Stir to make scrambled eggs.
9. Divide beans into 4 bowls. Add scrambled eggs. Top with tomato mix that you prepared at the beginning. Serve with your favorite salsa.

Enjoy!

Nutritional value: 236 calories, 14 grams of fat, 12 grams of carbs, 1 grams of fiber, 15 grams of protein

Special Cranberry Nut Bread

It's a perfect bread for a special breakfast!

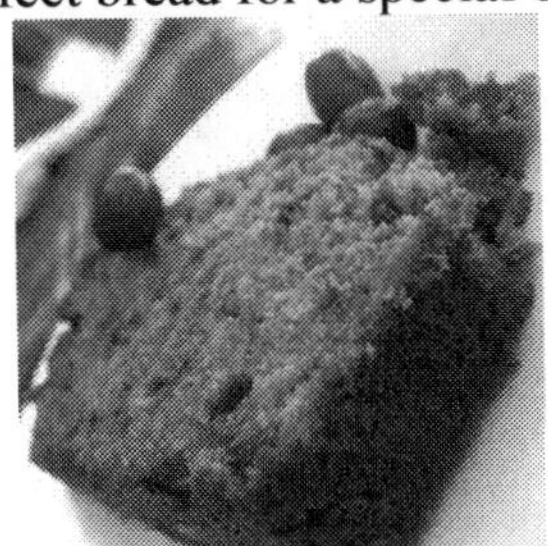

Ingredients:
2½ cups of almond flour
2 cups of whole cranberries
2½ teaspoons of baking powder
1/3 cup of powdered egg whites
A pinch of salt
1 cup of Splenda
3 eggs
¾ cup of water
1 stick of butter melted

Directions:

1. Grease a loaf pan with butter. Leave aside.
2. Put cranberries in your blender. Pulse them a few times.
3. In a bowl, mix almond flour with egg white powder, salt, and baking powder.
4. Add melted butter, Splenda, eggs, and water. Stir well.
5. Add cranberries. Stir. Pour into a loaf pan. Put in the oven. Bake at 350 degrees F for 50 minutes.
6. Take bread out of the oven. Leave it to cool down. Cut and serve.

Nutritional value: 164 calories, 2 grams of carbs, 2 grams of fiber, 6 grams of protein

Incredible Poppy Scones

These are some of the most delicious scones ever!

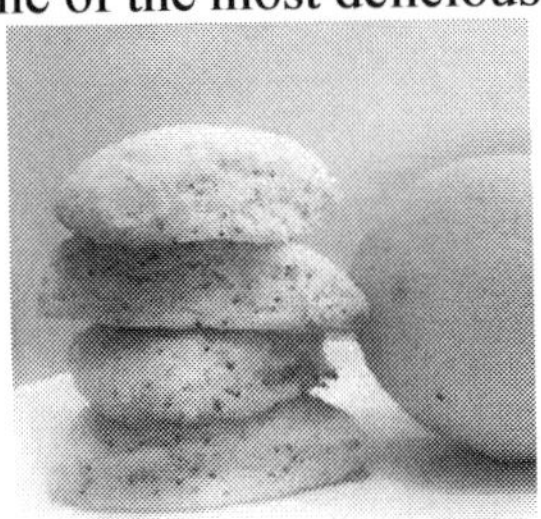

Ingredients:
2 cups of almond flour
¾ cup of Splenda
Zest and juice from 1 lemon
2 tablespoons of poppy seeds
A pinch of salt
4 teaspoons of baking powder
¾ cup of margarine
½ cup of soy milk
½ cup of water

Directions:

1. In a bowl, mix flour with salt and baking powder.
2. Add Splenda and margarine. Stir well.
3. Add lemon zest and juice, and poppy seeds. Stir again.
4. Add water and soy milk gradually to the mixture. Stir until you obtain a thick batter.
5. Grease a baking sheet with some butter. Make a scoop of about ¼ cup for each scone. Put in the oven at 400 degrees F. Bake for 15 minutes.
6. Take scones out of the oven. Leave them to cool down. Serve for breakfast!

Enjoy!

Nutritional value: 240 calories, 10 grams of fat, 20 grams of carbs, 0 grams of fiber, 5 grams of protein

Tasty Breakfast Potatoes

These potatoes are so good that they'll make you ask for more!

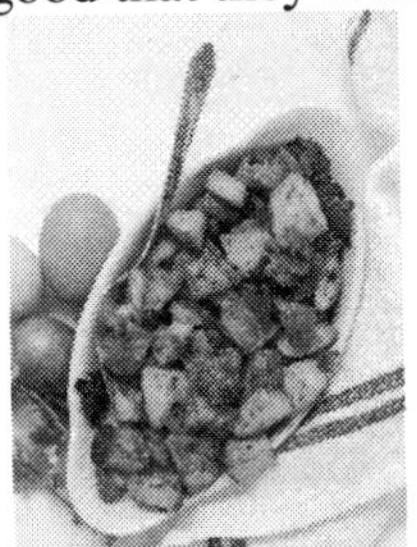

Ingredients:
2 pounds of potatoes, sliced evenly
½ white onion, sliced
1 red bell pepper, chopped
1 teaspoon of garlic powder
2 tablespoons of extra-virgin olive oil
Sea salt and black pepper to taste

Directions:

1. In a bowl, mix potatoes with onion and bell pepper.
2. Drizzle olive oil on top. Toss to coat.
3. Add salt, pepper, and garlic powder. Mix well.
4. Transfer everything onto a baking sheet. Put food in the oven at 425 degrees F. Bake for 45 minutes. Stir every 15 minutes.
5. Take potatoes out of the oven. Leave them to cool down. Transfer onto plates. Serve!

Enjoy!

Nutritional value: 160, 9 grams of fat, 20 grams of carbs, 3 grams of fiber, 3 grams of protein

Breakfast Oatmeal

This oatmeal is really something amazing!

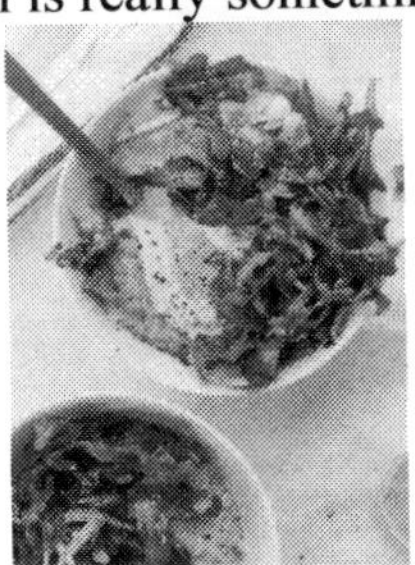

Ingredients:
1 cup of almond milk
3 cups of water
1 tablespoon of olive oil
1 cup of steel-cut oats
Salt and black pepper to taste
Some sundried tomatoes
4 poached eggs for serving

Directions:

1. Put water and almond milk in a pot. Bring to a boil. Simmer for a few minutes.
2. Meanwhile, heat up a pan with the olive oil at a medium temperature. Add oats. Stir and cook for 2 minutes.
3. Add oats to milk and water mixture. Stir. Reduce heat. Simmer for 25 minutes, stirring from time to time.
4. Add salt and pepper. Stir and simmer for 10 more minutes.
5. Remove from heat. Leave aside for 5 minutes. Add sun-dried tomatoes. Stir gently.
6. Pour into bowls. Top each one with poached eggs.
7. Serve hot!

Enjoy!

Nutritional value: 170 calories, 5 grams of fat, 10 grams of carbs, 1 gram of fiber, 3 grams of protein

Breakfast Tomato and Basil Quiche

It's a fancy breakfast that looks and tastes wonderful!

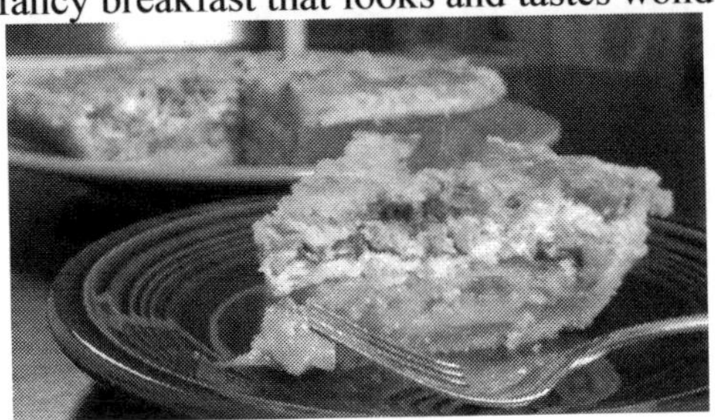

Ingredients:
3 eggs, whisked
1 tablespoon of extra-virgin olive oil
2 tomatoes, sliced
1 yellow onion, sliced
2 tablespoons of wholemeal flour
½ cup of almond milk
Salt and black pepper to taste
1 unbaked pie crust
2 teaspoons of basil
1½ cups of shredded cheese

Directions:

1. Put pie crust in the oven at 400 degrees F. Leave for 8 minutes. Take out of the oven. Leave aside for now.
2. Meanwhile, heat up a pan with the oil at a medium temperature. Cook onion slices for 5-6 minutes.
3. Remove onion from pan. Put in a bowl. Leave aside.
4. Mix tomato slices with flour and basil. Put them in the same heated pan. Sauté them for 1-2 minutes on each side. Transfer them into a bowl.
5. In a bowl, mix eggs with milk, salt, and pepper.
6. Spread 1 cup of shredded cheese on pie crust. Layer onion slices and tomato slices. Add egg mix at the end.
7. Sprinkle the rest of the cheese onto the pie. Put food in the oven at 400 degrees F. Bake for 10 minutes.
8. Reduce heat to 350 degrees F. Bake for 20 more minutes.
9. Take pie out of the oven. Leave it to cool down for a few minutes. Serve.

Enjoy!

Nutritional value: 238 calories, 13 grams of fat, 18 grams of carbs, 0 grams of fiber, 10 grams of protein

Breakfast Pumpkin Smoothie

It's perfect for pumpkin fans and it will make an autumn day a lot better!

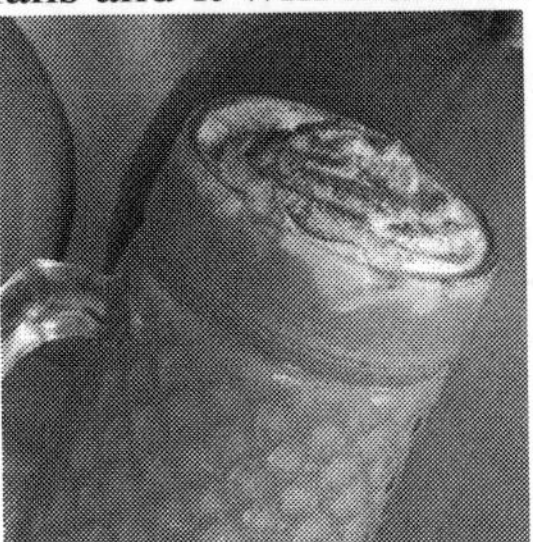

Ingredients:
16 ounces of already made pumpkin puree
2 cups of coconut water
2 teaspoons of cinnamon
¼ cup of Splenda

Directions:

1. Put pumpkin puree in a zip-top bag. Keep it in the freezer for 1 day.
2. Put puree in a bowl. Heat it up in your microwave for 2 minutes.
3. Pour coconut water into a blender. Add cinnamon and Splenda. Pulse a few times.
4. Add pumpkin puree. Blend again.
5. Pour into glasses. Serve!

Enjoy!

Nutritional value: 260 calories, 66 grams of carbs, 5 grams of protein, 1 gram of fat

Carrot Muffins

It's a splendid way to start a new day!

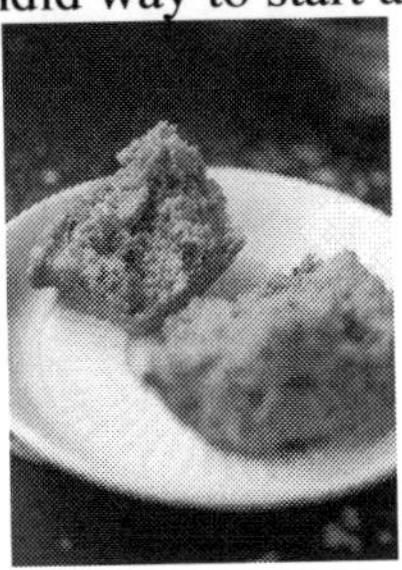

Ingredients:
1¾ cups of whole wheat flour
1 teaspoon of cinnamon
1½ teaspoons of baking powder
A pinch of salt
½ teaspoon of baking soda
½ teaspoon of ground ginger
2 cups of carrots, finely grated
¼ teaspoon of nutmeg
½ cup of raisins
½ cup of walnuts, roughly chopped
½ cup of coconut oil
2 eggs
½ cup of maple syrup
1 teaspoon of vanilla extract
Cooking spray

Directions:

1. Grease a muffin pan with some cooking spray. Leave aside for now.
2. In a bowl, mix flour with cinnamon, baking soda, baking powder, salt, ginger, and nutmeg. Stir well.
3. Add raisins, carrots and walnuts. Stir well.
4. In a bowl, mix oil with maple syrup. Add eggs. Whisk well.
5. Add vanilla extract at the end. Mix again.
6. Pour egg mixture into flour and carrots. Stir well.
7. Divide this batter into a muffin pan. Put food in the oven at 425 degrees F. Bake for 13 minutes.
8. Take muffins out of the oven. Leave them to cool down. Serve!

Enjoy!

Nutritional value: 300 calories, 6 grams of fat, 20 grams of carbs, 4 grams of fiber, 8 grams of protein

Tasty Aubergine and Pepper Pilaf

This wonderful recipe is full of rich nutrients and it's the best lunch idea ever!

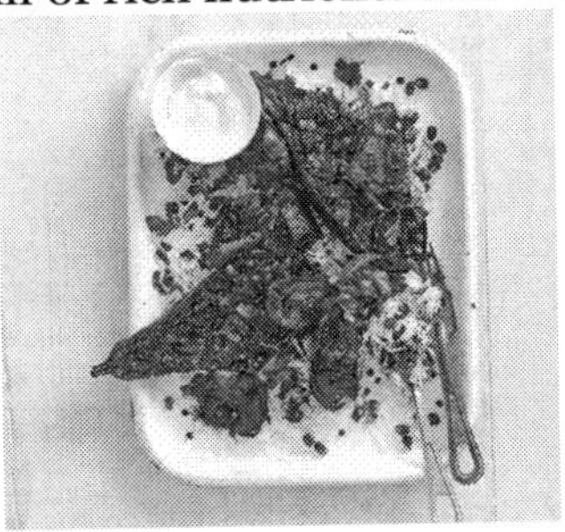

Ingredients:
2 tablespoons of extra-virgin olive oil
2 aubergines, cut in halves
2 red bell peppers, cut into quarters
2 teaspoons of chili flakes
2 teaspoons of cinnamon
2 teaspoons of za'atar
4 tablespoons of pomegranate molasses
5 ounces of lentils
5 ounces of basmati rice
Seeds from 1 pomegranate
A small handful of chopped parsley
Coconut yogurt for serving
Salt and black pepper to taste

Directions:

1. Prick aubergines with a fork. Brush them with 1 tablespoon of oil. Season with salt and pepper. Place on a baking tray. Put food in the oven at 350 degrees F. Bake for 15 minutes.
2. Take the tray out of the oven. Add peppers. Turn aubergines. Drizzle the rest of the oil.
3. Sprinkle cinnamon, chilies, za'atar, 1 tablespoon of pomegranate molasses. Put food back in the oven. Bake for 15 more minutes.
4. Meanwhile, put lentils in a pot with some water. Boil them at a medium-high temperature for 5 minutes.
5. Add rice. Cook for 10 minutes. Drain. Place back into the pot then add pomegranate seeds and parsley. Stir. Arrange on serving platters.
6. Take roasted vegetables out of the oven. Transfer them on top of lentils pilaf and the rice. Add coconut yogurt and the rest of the molasses on top. Serve!

Enjoy!

Nutritional value: 430 calories, 8 grams of fat, 70 grams of carbs, 16 grams of fibers, 16 grams of protein

Tasty Green Soup

It's a simple soup but with a unique taste! You should really consider making it!

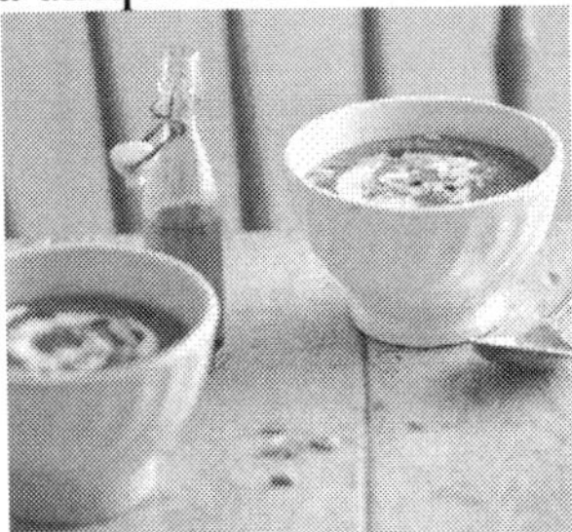

Ingredients:
1 yellow onion, finely chopped
2 garlic cloves, finely chopped
2 teaspoons of extra-virgin olive oil
1 medium potato, cubed
3 cups of vegetable stock
5 ounces of coconut yogurt
1 tablespoon of pine nuts, toasted
4 ounces of mixed watercress, spinach, and rocket
Chili oil for serving
Salt and black pepper to taste

Directions:

1. Heat up a pan with the oil at a medium-low temperature. Add onion, some salt and pepper. Cook for 10 minutes. Stir constantly.
2. Add garlic. Stir and cook for 1 more minute.
3. Add potato and the vegetable stock. Stir and simmer for 12 minutes.
4. Add salad mix. Cook for 1 minute. Take off heat. Blend using your food processor.
5. Transfer into serving bowl. Add some coconut yogurt, pine nuts and chili oil on top.

Enjoy!

Nutritional value: 320 calories, 12 grams of fat, 36 grams of carbs, 7 grams of fibers, 12 grams of protein

Delicious Cabbage and Fennel Seed Mix

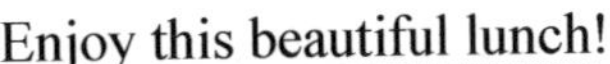
Enjoy this beautiful lunch!

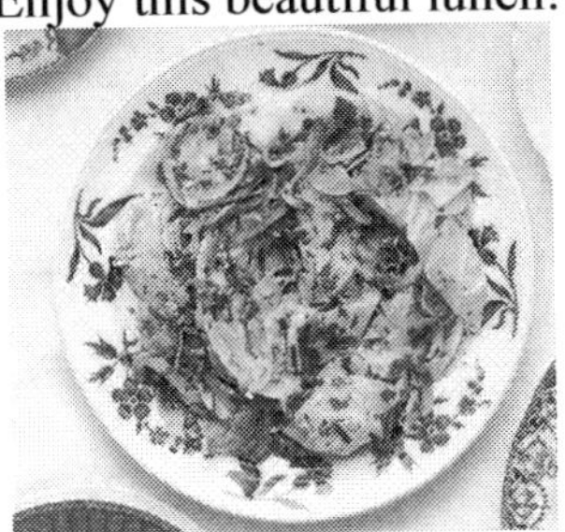

Ingredients:
1 large cabbage head, shredded
1 teaspoon of fennel seeds
2 tablespoons of olive oil
1 yellow onion, sliced
1 tablespoon of white wine vinegar
1 cup of dry white wine
½ of a small bunch of coriander, chopped
Salt and black pepper

Directions:

1. Heat up a pan with the oil, at a medium temperature. Add fennel seeds. Cook for 1 minute.
2. Add onion. Stir and cook for 2 minutes.
3. Add cabbage. Toss to coat. Cook for 2 minutes more.
4. Add vinegar and white wine. Stir and cook for 5 minutes.
5. Reduce heat. Simmer for 5 minutes.
6. Add coriander. Stir. Transfer onto plates. Serve!

Enjoy!

Nutritional value: 97 calories, 4 grams of fat, 5 grams of carbs, 3 grams of fibers, 2 grams of protein

Chili Bean Soup

A hearty soup for your next lunch!

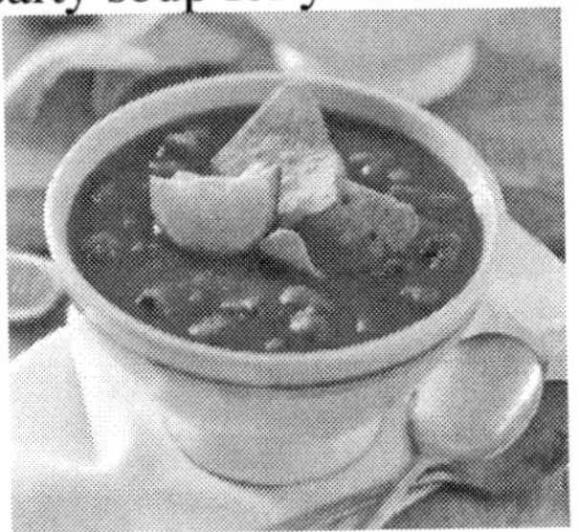

Ingredients:
1 yellow onion, finely chopped
1 tablespoon of extra-virgin olive oil
1 teaspoon of chili powder
1 tablespoon of tomato puree
1 garlic clove, crushed
½ teaspoon of cumin
Salt and black pepper to taste
14 ounces of canned tomatoes, chopped
1 red pepper, cut into chunks
13 ounces of canned mixed beans, drained
Tortilla chips for serving
½ can of water
4 lime wedges for serving

Directions:

1. Heat up a pan with the oil, at a medium temperature. Cook onion for 3-4 minutes.
2. Add tomato purée and garlic. Stir and cook for 2 minutes.
3. Add chili powder, cumin, salt and pepper. Cook for 1 minute.
4. Add tomatoes, water and stock. Simmer for 15 minutes.
5. Take off heat. Add more salt and pepper if needed. Blend soup using your food processor. Return to heat. Add beans and red pepper. Cook for 15 minutes more.
6. Transfer into a bowl. Serve with lime wedges and tortilla chips.

Enjoy!

Nutritional value: 157 calories, 4 grams of fat, 18 grams of carbs, 9 grams of fibers, 8 grams of protein

Indian Potato Dish

Why not try an Indian-style lunch for a change?

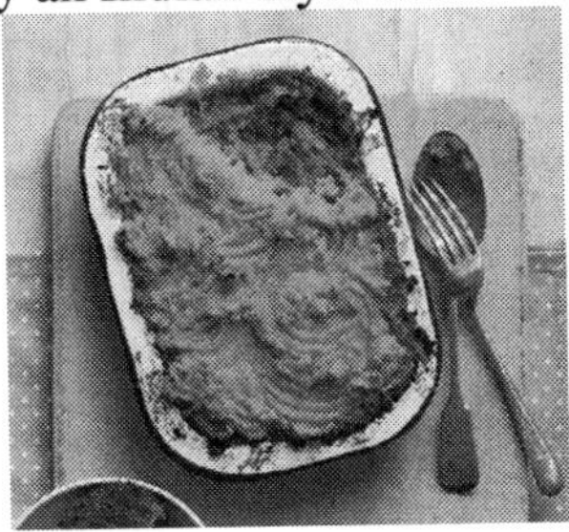

Ingredients:
22 ounces of sweet potatoes, cut into small chunks
2 carrots, sliced lengthwise
1 yellow onion, thinly sliced
1 teaspoon of grated ginger
2 garlic cloves, finely chopped
2 teaspoons of olive oil
1 vegetable stock cube
1 tablespoon of curry powder
Salt and pepper to taste
2 tablespoons of tomato puree
3 ounces of red lentils
3 cups of water
A handful of chopped coriander and some coriander sprigs for serving
2 tablespoons of coconut yogurt

Directions:

1. Put potatoes in a pan. Cover with water. Heat up to a medium-high temperature. Simmer for 15 minutes.
2. Meanwhile, heat up a pan with oil, at a medium-high temperature. Cook garlic and onion for 2 minutes.
3. Add carrots and ginger. Stir and cook for 2 more minutes.
4. Add curry powder. Stir well. Add stock cube mixed with 3 cups of water.
5. Also, add lentils and tomato puree. Cover pan. Boil for 20 minutes.
6. Add salt, pepper and coriander. Stir. Keep warm.
7. Drain potatoes. Mash them up. Mix with coconut yogurt.
8. Transfer lentils mix onto platters. Top with potato mash. Serve with coriander sprigs on top.

Enjoy!

Nutritional value: 450 calories, 4 grams of fat, 10 grams of carbs, 10 grams of fibers, 19 grams of protein

Special Barley Risotto

It's one vegetarian dish you won't ever forget!

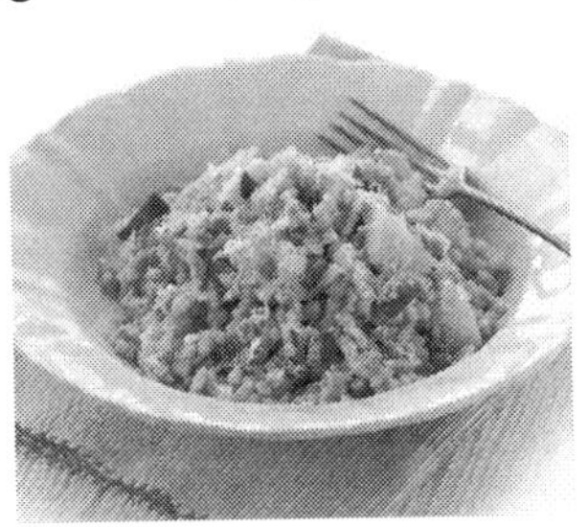

Ingredients:
1 tablespoon of melted butter
1 yellow onion, finely chopped
4 parsnips, cut into chunks
10 sage leaves, shredded
1 garlic clove, crushed
14 ounces of barley rinsed
½ tablespoon of grated parmesan cheese
6 cups of hot vegetable stock
Salt and black pepper

Directions:

1. Heat up a pan with the butter, at a medium-high temperature. Add onion and some salt and pepper. Cook for 5 minutes.
2. Add parsnips. Cook for 10 more minutes.
3. Add sage, garlic, and the barley. Stir well.
4. Add stock. Bring to a boil. Reduce heat. Simmer for 40 minutes.
5. Take the risotto off heat. Add parmesan. Stir. Transfer onto plates. Serve with black pepper and sage leaves on top.

Enjoy!

Nutritional value: 450 calories, 12 grams of fat, 10 grams of carbs, 13 grams of fibers, 15 grams of protein

Stuffed Squash

It's a fresh summer recipe, perfect for lunch!

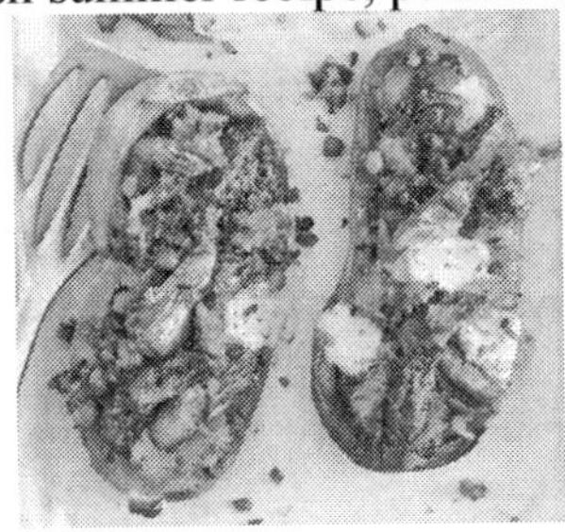

Ingredients:
1 butternut squash
1 ready-to-eat grain and chickpea pouch
4 ounces of artichokes in a jar
4 ounces of mozzarella and sun-dried tomato
Salt and black pepper to taste

Directions:

1. Cut squash in halves. Put into a heatproof bowl. Put in the microwave for 20 minutes. Take it out. Scoop flesh. Reserve the skin.
2. In a bowl, mix squash flesh with artichokes, grain and chickpea pouch, mozzarella and sun-dried tomato. Stir well.
3. Fill squash skin with this mix. Put food in the oven at 350 degrees F. Bake for 15 minutes.
4. Take out of the oven. Leave it to cool down. Serve right away!

Enjoy!

Nutritional value: 430 calories, 18 grams of fat, 55 grams of carbs, 14 grams of fibers, 16 grams of protein

Halloumi Salad

It's a great lunch idea!

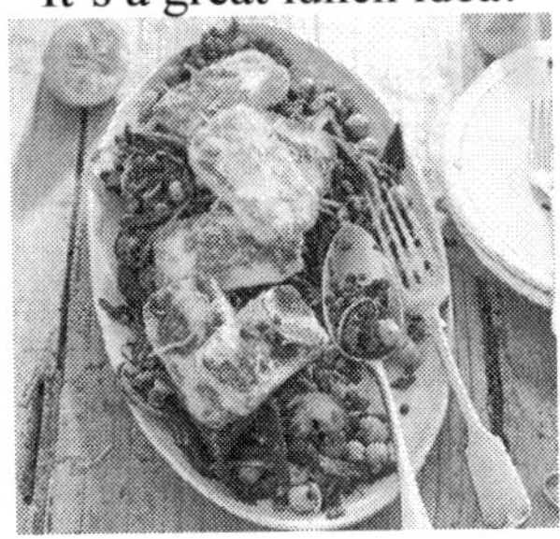

Ingredients:
7 ounces of lentils
3 tablespoons of chopped capers
Juice from 1 lemon
Zest and juice from 1 lemon
1 red onion sliced
3 tablespoons of olive oil
14 ounces of canned chickpeas, drained
8 ounces of already cooked beetroot, cut into matchsticks
1 small hand of parsley, finely chopped
8 ounces of packed halloumi, cut into 8 slices
Salt and pepper to taste

Directions:

1. Put lentils in a pot. Cover with water. Boil for 20 minutes. Drain. Leave aside.
2. Put lemon juice from 1 lemon in a bowl. Add onion, salt and pepper. Stir. Leave aside.
3. Put the juice and zest from the second lemon in a bowl. Add oil, salt, pepper and the capers. Stir well. Leave aside.
4. Put lentils and chickpeas in a bowl. Add beets, parsley and the pickled onions you prepared earlier. Toss to coat.
5. Heat up a grill at a medium temperature. Cook halloumi for 2 minutes on each side.
6. Add this to the salad. Add capers along with lemon juice and zest. Stir well. Serve.

Enjoy!
Nutritional value: 400 calories, 20 grams of fat, 20 grams of carbs, 12 grams of fibers, 13 grams of protein

Amazing Sweet Potatoes with Chickpeas Dish

It's one of the best vegetarian dishes you'll have!

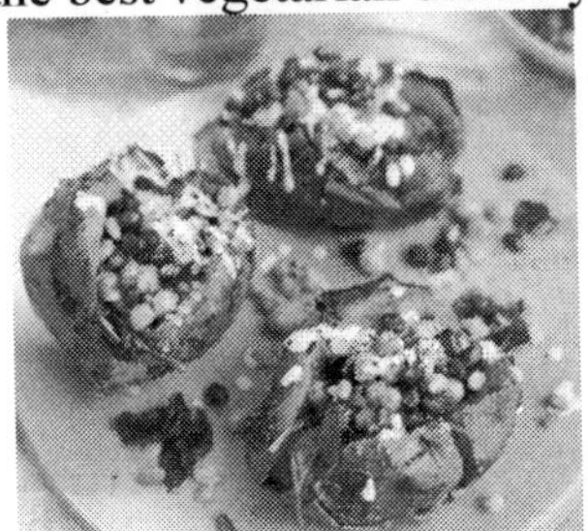

Ingredients:
4 tablespoons of olive oil
1 garlic clove, crushed
4 medium sweet potatoes
1 shallot, finely chopped
14 ounces of canned chickpeas, drained
3 ounces of baby spinach
Zest and juice from 1 lemon
A small bunch of dill, finely chopped
For the tahini yogurt:
1½ tablespoons of coconut yogurt
½ tablespoon of pine nuts
2 tablespoons of tahini
4 ounces of pomegranate seeds
Salt and pepper to taste

Directions:

1. Wrap potatoes in tin foil. Arrange on a baking sheet. Put food in the oven at 350 degrees F. Cook for 1 hour.
2. Meanwhile, heat up a pan with 1 tablespoon of olive oil, at a medium-high temperature. Cook shallot and garlic for 3 minutes.
3. Add chickpeas. Stir and cook for 1 more minute.
4. Add spinach and dill. Stir. Take off heat. Leave aside.
5. In a bowl, mix the rest of the oil with lemon zest and juice. Stir.
6. Add salt and pepper to chickpea mix. Mash everything with a potato masher.
7. In another bowl, mix coconut yogurt with tahini, salt, and pepper. Stir well.
8. Take potatoes out of the oven. Unwrap them. Split them lengthwise. Put on plates. Fill with chickpea mix. Drizzle tahini mix over them. Serve with pine nuts and pomegranate seeds on top.

Enjoy!

Nutritional value: 400 calories, 23 grams of fat, 45 grams of carbs, 13 grams of fibers, 12 grams of protein

Delicious Poached Potatoes

It's a flavored dish!

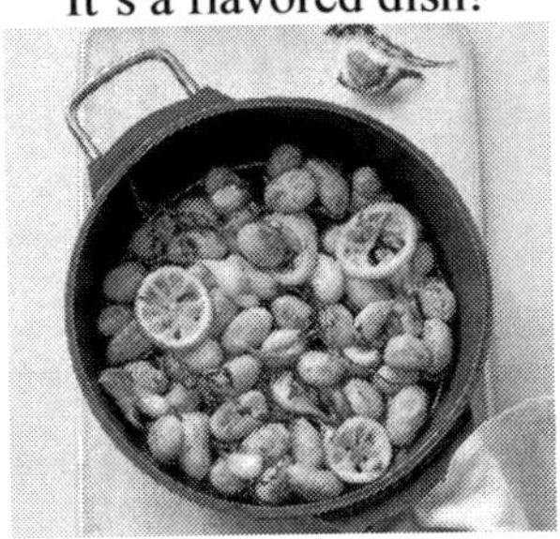

Ingredients:
21 ounces of sweet potatoes
2 garlic heads, divided into cloves
1 teaspoon of black peppercorns
1 lemon, sliced
3 thyme sprigs
1 teaspoon of chopped thyme
10 ounces of rapeseed oil
Salt and black pepper to taste

Directions:

1. In an oven-proof dish, add peppercorns, potatoes, lemon slices, garlic, thyme sprigs, salt, pepper and the oil.
2. Toss to coat. Cover. Put food in the oven at 360 degrees F. Bake for 45 minutes.
3. Take the dish out of the oven. Leave it to cool down for 20 minutes. Transfer onto plates. Serve with chopped thyme on top.

Enjoy!

Nutritional value: 250 calories, 17 grams of fat, 20 grams of carbs, 4 grams of proteins, 4 grams of fibers

Vegetable Dish

It's quick and tastes wonderful!

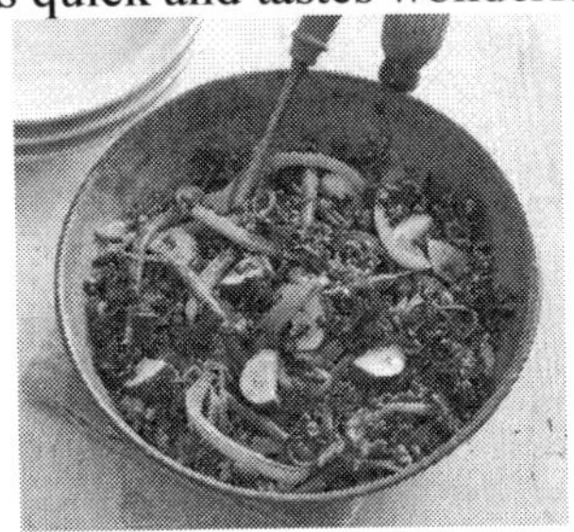

Ingredients:
1½ tablespoons of tahini
1½ tablespoons of water
Juice and zest of 1 lemon
2 tablespoons of extra-virgin olive oil
1 garlic clove, crushed
1 red onion, thinly sliced
1 yellow pepper, thinly sliced
1 courgette, sliced
7 ounces of green beans halved
8 ounces of pre-cooked lentils
3 ounces of kale, shredded
Salt and black pepper to taste

Directions:

1. In a bowl, mix lemon zest and juice with tahini. Stir well.
2. Add water, salt and pepper. Stir to obtain a dressing. Leave aside.
3. Heat up a pan with the oil, at a medium-high temperature. Cook onion with a pinch of salt, for 2 minutes.
4. Add green pepper, garlic, green beans and courgette. Cook for 5 minutes. Stir constantly.
5. Add kale, lentils, and the tahini dressing. Cook for 2-3 minutes more.
6. Take off heat. Transfer onto plates. Serve hot!

Enjoy!

Nutritional value: 240 calories, 14 grams of fat, 23 grams of carbs, 10 grams of fibers, 13 grams of protein

Asparagus and Potato Frittata

It's a simple lunch idea, ready to eat in no time!

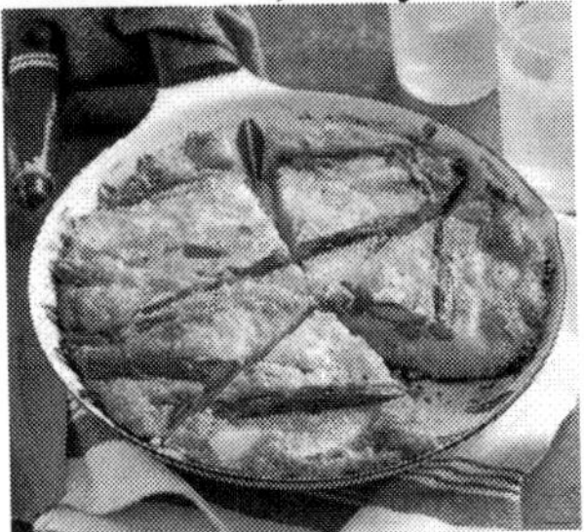

Ingredients:
1 tablespoon of olive oil
1 yellow onion, finely chopped
7 ounces of potatoes, cut in quarters
4 ounces of asparagus tips
6 eggs, whisked
1 tablespoon of cheddar cheese, grated
Some mixed leaves for serving
Salt and black pepper to taste

Directions:

1. Put potatoes in a pot. Cover with water. Add some salt. Bring to a boil. Leave them to cook for 5 minutes. Add asparagus. Leave for 1 more minute. Take off heat. Drain. Leave aside for now.
2. Heat up a pan with the oil, at a medium-high temperature. Cook onion for 8 minutes.
3. In a bowl, mix eggs with salt, pepper, and half of the cheese. Stir.
4. Add eggs to the onion. Add asparagus and potatoes as well. Top with the rest of the cheese. Cook for 5-6 minutes.
5. Take frittata off heat. Cut into wedges. Serve with mixed leaves on the side.

Enjoy!

Nutritional value: 300 calories, 18 grams of fat, 16 grams of carbs, 4 grams of fibers, 19 grams of protein

Special Surprise Dish

An amazing dish to try!

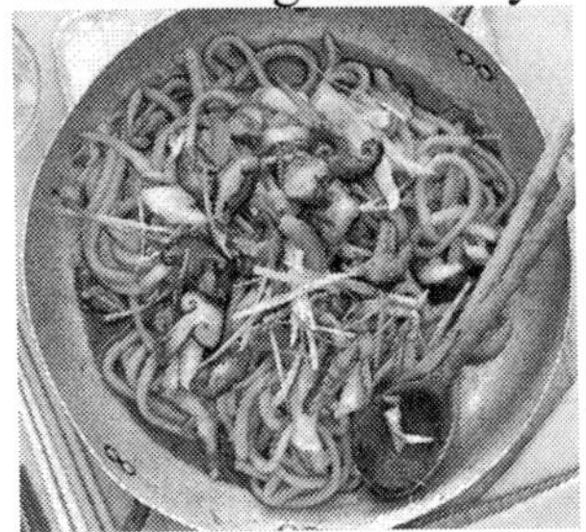

Ingredients:
9 ounces of dried udon noodles
9 ounces of cold water
1 yellow onion, thickly sliced
2 tablespoons of sesame oil
10 shitake mushrooms
¼ head cabbage, roughly chopped
4 spring onions, finely sliced
Salt and black pepper to taste
For the sauce:
2 tablespoons of soy sauce
4 tablespoons of mirin
1 tablespoon of Worcestershire sauce
A pinch of Stevia

Directions:

1. Put some water into a pot. Bring to a boil. Add 9 ounces of cold water and the noodles. Cook for 5 minutes. Drain. Leave aside.
2. Heat up a pan with 1 tablespoon of oil. Add onion and cabbage. Cook for 5 minutes.
3. Add mushrooms and spring onions. Cook for 1 more minute.
4. Add the noodles, salt, pepper and the rest of the oil. Stir. Keep on the stove for 1-2 more minutes.
5. In a bowl, mix Worcestershire sauce with Stevia, soy sauce, and mirin. Stir. Add to noodle mix.
6. Toss to coat. Take off heat. Serve!

Enjoy!

Nutritional value: 400 calories, 14 grams of fat, 70 grams of carbs, 10 grams of fibers, 12 grams of protein

Asparagus and Courgette Salad

It's a flavored salad that will transform your lunch into a real feast!

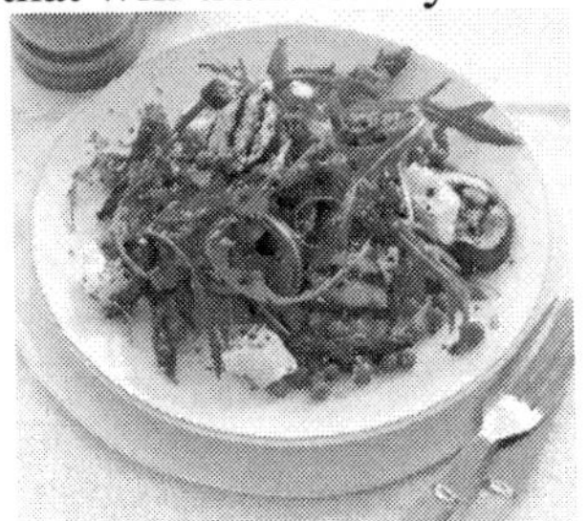

Ingredients:
1½ tablespoons of peas
1 teaspoon of sesame seed
5 ounces of asparagus
1 teaspoon of sesame oil
7 ounces of courgettes, sliced
A handful of rocket leaves
1 tablespoon of feta cheese, grated
Zest from ½ of a lemon
Salt and black pepper to taste

Directions:

1. Heat up a pan at a medium-high temperature. Add sesame seeds. Toast them for 1-2 minutes. Take off heat. Leave aside.
2. Steam asparagus for 3-4 minutes. Transfer them into a bowl filled with ice water. Drain. Leave aside.
3. Put peas in a pot filled with water. Bring to a boil. Cook for 3 minutes.
4. Drain. Leave aside as well.
5. Heat up a grill. Brush asparagus and courgette slices with oil. Cook them for a few minutes.
6. Transfer courgette slices and asparagus into a bowl. Add peas, rocket, feta and lemon zest.
7. Add salt and black pepper. Sprinkle sesame seeds on top.

Enjoy!

Nutritional value: 214 calories, 11 grams of fat, 12 grams of carbs, 9 grams of fibers, 15 grams of protein

Tasty Pepper and Bean Salad

It's a super easy and quick lunch idea!

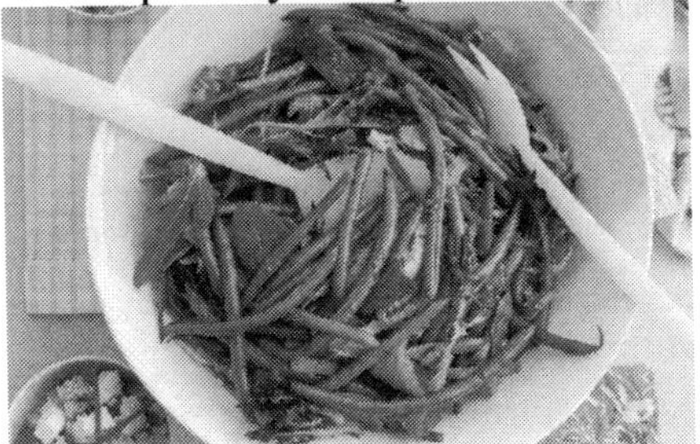

Ingredients:
2 yellow peppers, deseeded and cut into halves
2 red peppers, deseeded and cut into halves
17 ounces of green beans
7 ounces of salad leaves
For the dressing:
2 tablespoons of balsamic vinegar
6 tablespoons of extra-virgin olive oil
1 tablespoon of grated ginger

Directions:

1. Place all peppers onto a baking tray. Put them in the oven. Bake at 400 degrees F for 20 minutes. Remove food from the oven. Place in a zip-top bag. Leave them to cool down. Peel the skin. Chop. Place in a bowl. Leave aside.
2. Meanwhile, place beans in a pot filled with boiling water. Cook for 5 minutes at a medium-high temperature. Drain. Leave aside to cool down.
3. Mix beans with peppers and salad in a large salad bowl.
4. In another bowl, mix olive oil with vinegar and ginger. Stir well.
5. Add this dressing to the salad. Toss to coat. Serve right away.

Enjoy!

Nutritional value: 123 calories, 5 grams of fat, 10 grams of carbs, 7 grams of fibers, 12 grams of protein

Tasty Potato Soup

Eat a tasty soup for lunch and you will get all the energy you need for the rest of the day!

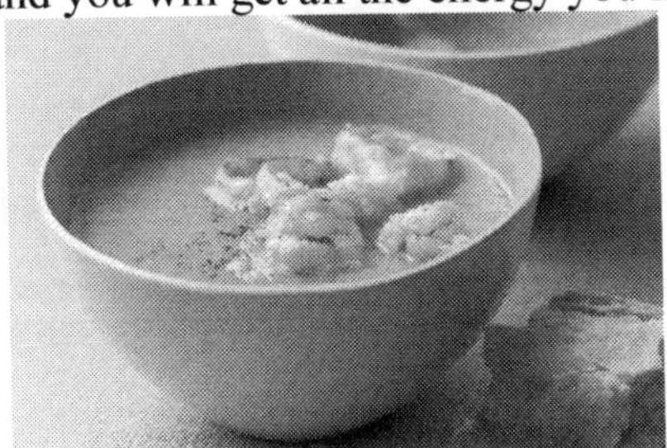

Ingredients:
2 large leeks, sliced
1 yellow onion, chopped
½ tablespoon of butter
2 vegetable stock cubes
1 large potato, peeled and chopped
4 ounces of peas
Salt and pepper to taste
For the garnish:
A pinch of saffron threads
Some leek slices
1 egg white
1 tablespoon of almond flour
Vegetable oil for frying
35 ounces of water

Directions:

1. Heat up a pot with butter, at a medium-high temperature. Cook leeks and onion for 10 minutes. Stir constantly.
2. Add water and stock cubes. Bring to a boil. Add potato. Cook for 10 minutes.
3. Add peas. Cook for 10 more minutes
4. Meanwhile, in a bowl, mix egg white with saffron. Whisk well.
5. Add flour, salt and pepper to taste. Stir again well.
6. Heat up a pan with the oil, at a medium-high temperature. Dip leek slices in the batter you've prepared. Place them in the heated pan. Fry them until they become golden.
7. Drain excess grease from fried leeks using paper towels. Leave aside for now.
8. Take soup off the heat. Pour into your food processor. Season with salt and pepper. Blend well.
9. Pour soup into serving bowls. Add leek rings on top. Serve.

Enjoy!

Nutritional value: 130 calories, 6 grams of fat, 15 grams of carbs, 7 grams of fibers, 16 grams of protein

Easy Vegetable Dish

It's one vegetable dish you'll adore!

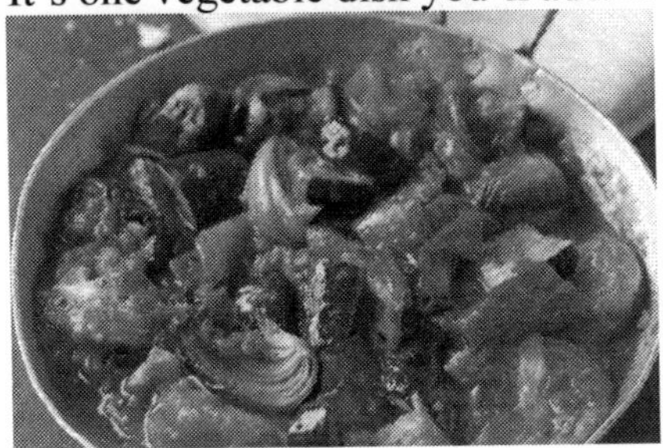

Ingredients:
1 aubergine, thickly sliced (each slice cut in halves)
2 bell peppers, cut into large chunks
2 courgettes, halved and cut into large chunks
4 plum tomatoes, halved
2 red onions, cut into wedges
1 tablespoon of oregano
5 tablespoons of extra-virgin olive oil
Salt and black pepper to taste
2 garlic cloves, finely chopped
14 ounces of canned tomatoes, chopped

Directions:

1. Make a single layer of aubergine slices in a baking pan.
2. Add bell peppers, courgettes, tomatoes and red onions.
3. Add oregano, salt, black pepper and 4 tablespoons of olive oil. Toss everything to coat.
4. Put food in the oven at 375 degrees F. Bake for 45 minutes. Stir from time to time.
5. Heat up a pan with the rest of the olive oil, at a medium-high temperature. Cook the garlic for 2-3 minutes.
6. Add canned tomatoes. Bring to a boil. Cook for 10 minutes.
7. Add this to the vegetables. Stir gently. Transfer onto serving plates. Serve while it's hot.

Enjoy!

Nutritional value: 150 calories, 3 grams of fat, 16 grams of carbs, 13 grams of fibers, 15 grams of protein

Mushroom Gratin

It's one of the best vegetarian dishes you could have!

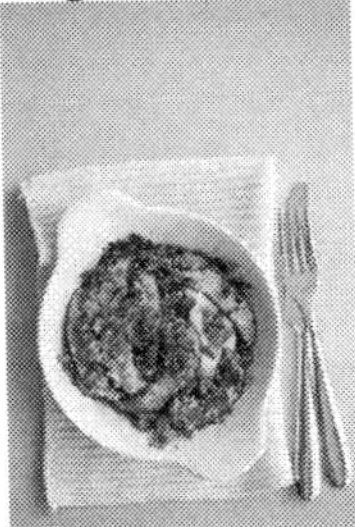

Ingredients:
1 large Portobello mushroom, sliced
1 tablespoon of water
½ tablespoon of breadcrumbs
1 teaspoon of olive oil
Salt and black pepper to taste
1 teaspoon of chives, chopped

Directions:

1. Put mushroom slices in a baking dish. Add water. Drizzle oil. Season with salt and pepper. Sprinkle breadcrumbs on top.
2. Place dish on a grill. Cook for 10 minutes.
3. Take off heat. Sprinkle chives on top. Serve.

Enjoy!

Nutritional value: 90 calories, 3 grams of fat, 10 grams of carbs, 7 grams of protein, 5 grams of fibers

Tasty Tuscan Soup

It's a traditional Tuscan soup, perfect for fasting days!

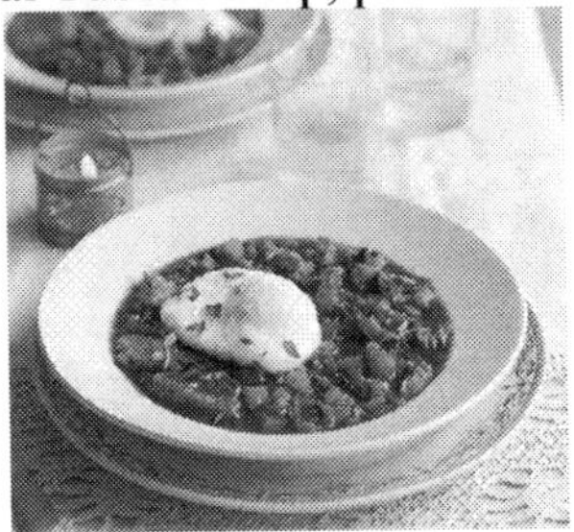

Ingredients:
3 tablespoons of extra-virgin olive oil
2 carrots, chopped
3 celery stick, chopped
2 garlic cloves, chopped
1 red onion, chopped
2 teaspoons of thyme, chopped
1½ tablespoons of dried porcini mushrooms
8 ounces of plum tomatoes chopped
4 cups of chicken stock
2 tablespoons of parsley, chopped
3 slices of toasted bread, cut into chunks
6 poached eggs

Directions:

1. Heat up a saucepan with the oil, at a medium-high temperature. Cook celery, onion, carrots, thyme and garlic for 15 minutes. Stir occasionally.
2. Put mushrooms in a bowl. Cover them with hot water. Leave aside for 15 minutes.
3. Drain them. Reserve liquid. Chop. Add mushrooms to the vegetables.
4. Also, add reserved liquid. Stir. Cook for 5 minutes.
5. Add tomatoes. Cook for 10 minutes. Add the stock.
6. Bring to a simmer. Cook for another 5-6 minutes.
7. Pour into serving bowls. Add toasted bread. Top with poached eggs. Sprinkle parsley.

Enjoy!

Nutritional value: 220 calories, 6 grams of fat, 13 grams of carbs, 6 grams of fibers, 16 grams of protein

Eggs and Chips

Everyone loves this dish!

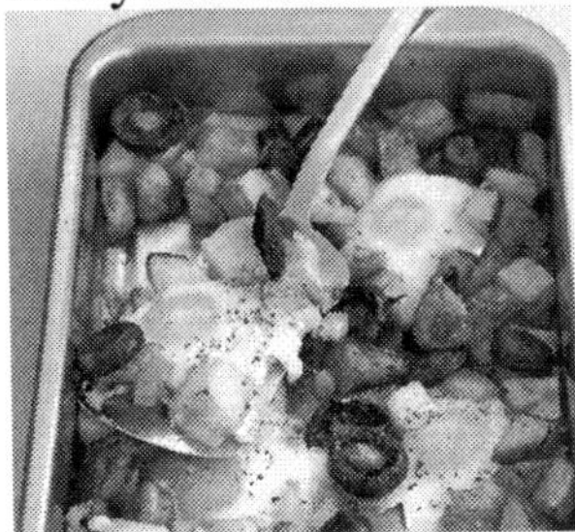

Ingredients:
17 ounces of potatoes, sliced
1 tablespoon of extra-virgin olive oil
2 shallots, sliced
2 teaspoons of oregano
7 ounces of mushrooms, chopped
4 eggs

Directions:

1. Place potatoes and shallots into a baking dish.
2. Drizzle oil on top. Add oregano. Mix well.
3. Put food in the oven at 350 degrees F. Bake for 45 minutes.
4. Take out of the oven. Add mushrooms. Bake for 10 more minutes.
5. Take out of the oven again. Make 4 gaps into the vegetables. Crack eggs. Put in the oven again. Cook for 4 minutes more.
6. Transfer onto plates. Serve right away!

Enjoy!

Nutritional value: 240 calories, 7 grams of fat, 7 grams of carbs, 10 grams of protein, 6 grams of fiber

Spicy Butternut Soup

A delicious, low-calorie soup.

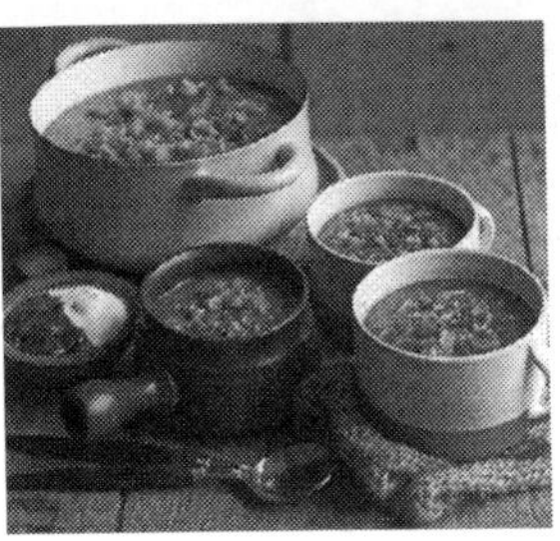

Ingredients:
2 yellow onions, finely chopped
2 tablespoons of extra-virgin olive oil
1 peeled apple, finely chopped
½ butternut squash, peeled and chopped
3 celery sticks, chopped
3 tablespoons of gluten-free curry powder
1 tablespoon of nigella seeds
1 tablespoon of cinnamon
Salt and black pepper to taste
28 ounces of canned tomatoes, chopped
7 cups of chicken stock
5 ounces of basmati rice
A small bunch of parsley, chopped
3 tablespoons of mango chutney

Directions:

1. Heat up a pot with the oil, at a medium-high temperature. Add apples, celery, onions and a pinch of salt. Stir and cook for 10 minutes.
2. Add squash, cinnamon, curry powder, nigella seeds, and some black pepper. Stir and cook for 2 more minutes.
3. Add tomatoes and chicken stock. Cover. Boil for 15 minutes.
4. Add rice. Cover again. Boil for 12 more minutes.
5. Add more salt and pepper, parsley and mango chutney. Stir gently.
6. Pour into bowls.

Enjoy!

Nutritional value: 240 calories, grams of fats 7, 12 grams of carbs, 10 grams of protein, 6 grams of fiber

Mushroom Pilaf

It's much lighter than a risotto and it tastes so good!

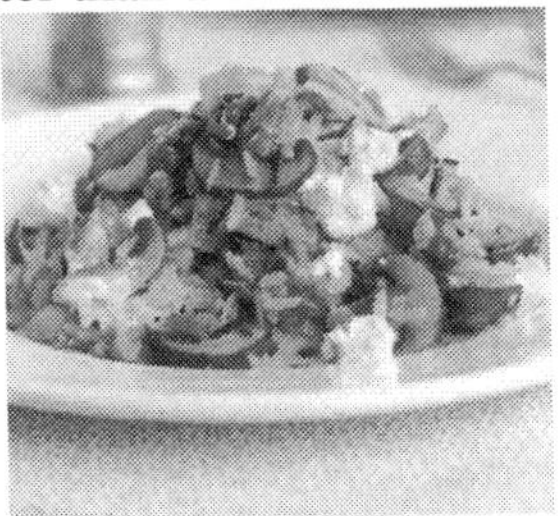

Ingredients:
2 cups of chicken stock
1 yellow onion, chopped
10 ounces of mixed mushrooms, sliced
2 garlic cloves, chopped
8 ounces of wild and basmati rice
Juice and zest of 1 lemon
A small bunch of chives, finely chopped
6 tablespoons of light goat cheese with herbs
Salt and black pepper to taste

Directions:

1. Heat up 2 tablespoons of stock in a pot at a medium-high temperature. Cook the onion for 5 minutes. Stir occasionally.
2. Add more stock and the mushrooms and garlic. Cook for 2 more minutes.
3. Add rice, lemon juice, lemon zest, salt, pepper and the rest of the stock.
4. Bring to a boil. Cover pot. Reduce heat. Simmer for 25 minutes.
5. Add half of the chives and half of the cheese. Stir gently.
6. Take off heat. Transfer onto plates. Serve with the rest of the chives sprinkled on top and with the rest of the cheese.

Enjoy!

Nutritional value: 170 calories, 7 grams of fat, 8 grams of carbs, 14 grams of protein, 2 grams of fiber

Potato Tortilla

A Spanish dish for your next lunch!

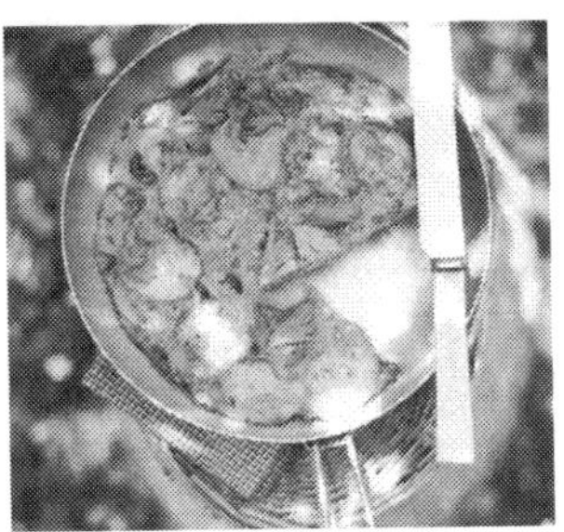

Ingredients:
9 ounces of potatoes, thickly sliced
3 tablespoons of extra-virgin olive oil
1 yellow onion, sliced
2 garlic cloves, chopped
½ teaspoons of smoked paprika
3 tablespoons of parsley, chopped
6 eggs
Salt and black pepper to taste

Directions:

1. Heat up a pan with oil, at a medium-high temperature. Fry potatoes for 3-4 minutes.
2. Add onion and garlic. Stir and cook for 7 more minutes.
3. Add paprika. Stir and cook for 1 minute more.
4. Meanwhile, in a bowl, whisk eggs well. Add salt, pepper and parsley. Stir.
5. Pour eggs over potatoes. Stir gently. Reduce heat. Cook for 10 minutes.
6. Transfer onto a plate. Sprinkle some parsley on top. Serve!

Enjoy!

Nutritional value: 180 calories, 2 grams of fat, 6 grams of carbs, 15 grams of protein, 10 grams of fiber

Delicious Potatoes and Black Beans

A perfect lunch recipe for a cold autumn day!

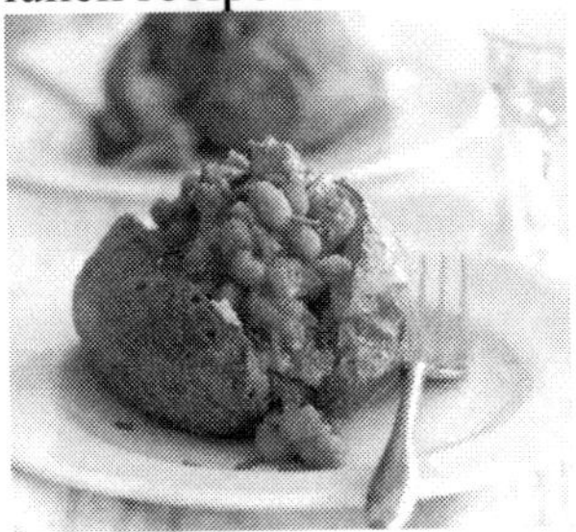

Ingredients:
4 large potatoes
1 carrot, chopped
1 tablespoon of sunflower oil
1 celery stalk, chopped
2 tomatoes, chopped
A splash of water
1 teaspoon of sweet paprika
14 ounces of canned haricot beans, drained
1 teaspoon of Worcestershire sauce
Salt and black pepper to taste
2 tablespoons of chives, chopped for serving

Directions:

1. Scrub potatoes. Dry them using paper towels. Prick them with a fork. Put food in the oven. Bake at 350 degrees F for 1 hour.
2. Meanwhile, heat up the oil in a pan at a medium-high temperature. Cook celery and carrot for 10 minutes.
3. Add beans, tomatoes, salt, pepper and sweet paprika. Stir and cook for 5 more minutes.
4. Add a splash of water and a small amount of Worcestershire sauce. Stir and cook for 5 minutcs.
5. Take off heat. Keep warm for now.
6. Take potatoes out of the oven. Split them. Spoon bean mix into them. Sprinkle chives on top. Arrange potatoes on plates. Serve.

Enjoy!

Nutritional value: 225 calories, 4 grams of fat, 7 grams of carbs, 14 grams of proteins, 6 grams of fiber

Beetroot Salad

You don't need only fancy dishes for lunch! Why shouldn't you enjoy a tasty salad instead?

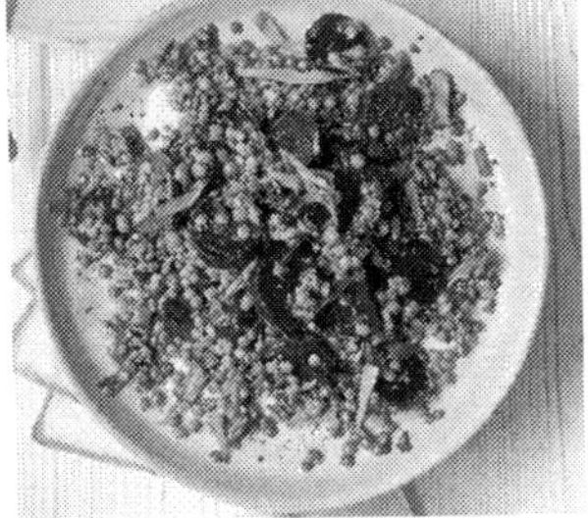

Ingredients:
7 ounces of pre-cooked lentils
1 tablespoon of wholegrain mustard
1½ tablespoon of extra-virgin olive oil
8 ounces of packed already cooked beetroot, sliced
A handful of tarragon, chopped
Salt and black pepper to taste

Directions:

1. In a bowl, mix mustard with oil, salt, and pepper. Stir well. Leave aside for now.
2. In a salad bowl, mix lentils with beetroot.
3. Add dressing. Toss to coat. Season some more. Sprinkle tarragon. Serve.

Enjoy!

Nutritional value: 150 calories, 5 grams of fat, 10 grams of carbs, 14 grams of proteins, 7 grams of fiber

Kale Salad

A healthy combination of ingredients!

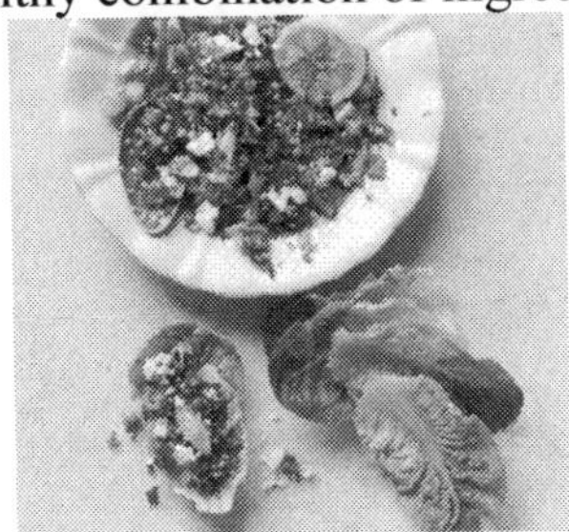

Ingredients:
4 ounces of bulgur wheat
4 ounces of kale
A bunch of mint, chopped
A bunch of spring onions, chopped
½ cucumber, chopped
A pinch of cinnamon
A pinch of allspice
6 tablespoons of extra-virgin olive oil
Zest and juice from ½ lemon
4 ounces of feta cheese, crumbled
4 heads of Baby Gem lettuce for serving

Directions:

1. Put bulgur in a bowl. Cover with boiling water. Leave aside for 10 minutes.
2. Put kale through the food processor.
3. Drain bulgur. Put in a bowl. Mix with kale, mint, spring onions, cucumber and tomatoes.
4. Add cinnamon and allspice. Stir.
5. Add olive oil and lemon juice. Toss to coat.
6. Add feta cheese and lemon zest on top
7. Arrange lettuce leaves on plates. Scoop salad into each.

Enjoy!

Nutritional value: 200 calories, 9 grams of fat, 12 grams of carbs, 14 grams of protein, 6 grams of fiber

Delightful Stuffed Marrow

Are you in the mood for something different? Then, instead of using courgettes, try using marrows!

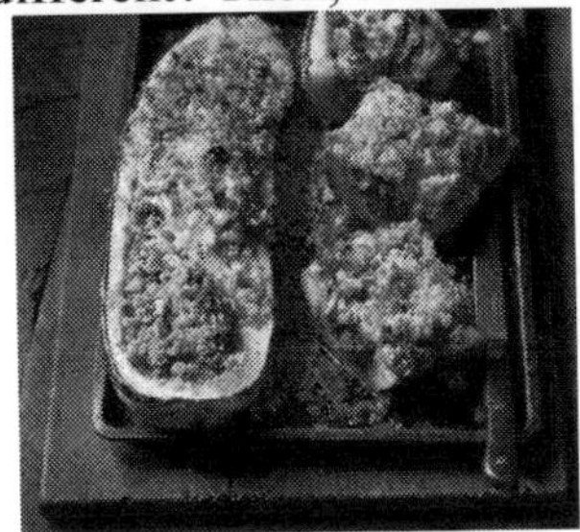

Ingredients:
1 marrow
1 yellow onion, chopped
1 tablespoon of extra-virgin olive oil
2 garlic cloves, crushed
4 ounces of chorizo, chopped
½ teaspoons of cayenne pepper
1 teaspoon of smoked paprika
½ teaspoon of dried oregano
½ teaspoon of dried thyme
28 ounces of canned chopped tomatoes
5 ounces of jarred roasted red pepper, sliced
A handful of parsley, chopped
2 tablespoons of breadcrumbs
4 ounces of grated cheese
Salt and pepper to taste

Directions:

1. Cut marrow in half lengthwise. Take the middle out. Arrange in a baking dish. Season with salt and pepper. Leave aside.
2. Heat up a pan with the oil, at a medium temperature. Cook the onion for 10 minutes.
3. Add garlic, chorizo, cayenne pepper, paprika, oregano, and thyme. Stir. Lower heat. Cook for another 2-3 minutes.
4. Add parsley, tomatoes and peppers. Stir and cook for 8-9 minutes more.
5. Fill each marrow half with this mixture. Cover the dish with tin foil. Put food in the oven at 350 degrees F. Bake for 30 minutes.
6. Take the dish out of the oven. Sprinkle breadcrumbs and cheese. Bake for 10 more minutes.
7. Take the marrow out of the oven. Leave it to cool down for a few minutes. Then serve.

Enjoy!

Nutritional value: 250 calories, 10 grams of fat, 15 grams of carbs, 14 grams of proteins, 6 grams of fiber

Stuffed Peppers

It's going to be one of the best vegetable dishes you'll ever have!

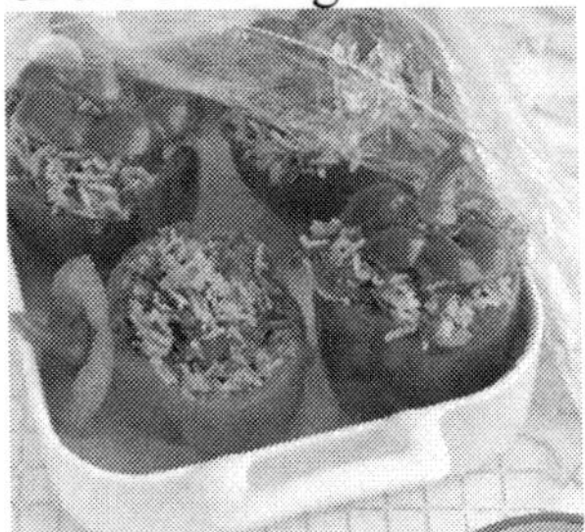

Ingredients:
2 garlic cloves, crushed
1 tablespoon of vegetable oil
1 yellow onion, chopped
1 small piece of ginger, finely chopped
1 teaspoon of cumin
1 teaspoon of tomato puree
1 teaspoon of garam masala
7 ounces of basmati rice
3½ cups of vegetable stock
5 ounces of red lentils
7 ounces of bag spinach leaves, chopped
8 bell peppers
Salt and black pepper to taste

Directions:

1. Heat up a saucepan with the oil, at a medium-high temperature. Cook onion, ginger and garlic for 5 minutes.
2. Add tomato puree, garam masala, cumin, salt, and pepper. Stir and cook for 1 more minutes.
3. Add rice and stock. Stir. Bring to a boil.
4. Add lentils. Cover. Reduce heat to low. Cook for 15 minutes.
5. Add spinach and mint. Stir well.
6. Meanwhile, cut the top of each pepper. Get the middle and the seeds out. Trim the bottoms and fill them with the rice and lentil mix. Arrange in a baking dish. Cover. Put food in the oven at 360 degrees F. Bake for 30 minutes.
7. Take out of the oven. Transfer peppers onto plates. Serve with some Greek yogurt on top.

Enjoy!

Nutritional value: 160 calories, 3 grams of fat, 5 grams of carbs, 10 grams of proteins, 9 grams of fiber

Bean Tostadas

Try this Mexican style lunch!

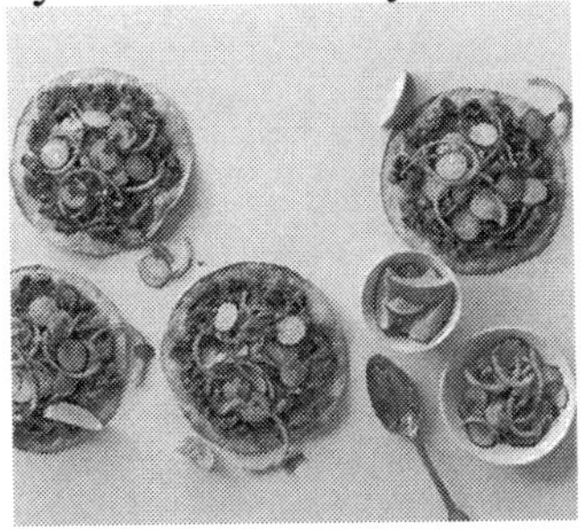

Ingredients:
1 red onion, thinly sliced
1 red onion, finely chopped
Juice from 1 lime
1 lime cut into wedges
1½ tablespoon of olive oil
2 teaspoons of cumin
2 garlic cloves, chopped
1 tablespoon of chipotle paste
1 tablespoon of tomato purée
14 ounces of canned kidney beans, drained and rinsed
4 corn tortillas
A sprigs coriander, chopped
5 ounces of radish, thinly sliced
Salt and black pepper to taste

Directions:

1. In a bowl, mix sliced onion with lime juice, salt, and pepper. Stir. Leave aside.
2. Meanwhile, heat up a pan with 1 tablespoon of oil, at a medium-high temperature. Cook chopped onion and garlic for a few minutes.
3. Add cumin. Stir and cook for 1 minute.
4. Add chipotle paste, tomato puree and beans. Stir.
5. Add some water. Stir and boil for 5 minutes.
6. Take off heat. Add salt and pepper. Mash everything.
7. Meanwhile, arrange tortillas on a baking sheet. Brush them with the rest of the sunflower oil. Put food in the oven at 350 degrees. Bake for 8 minutes.
8. Take tortillas out of the oven. Arrange on a platter. Spread the bean puree you prepared earlier.
9. In a bowl, mix radishes with coriander and the pickled onions.
10. Spread this over the bean mixture. Serve with lime wedges.

Enjoy!

Nutritional value: 230 calories, 6 grams of fat, 8 grams of carbs, 3 grams of protein, 10 grams of fiber

Tomato Soup

This Mediterranean-style soup tastes wonderful!

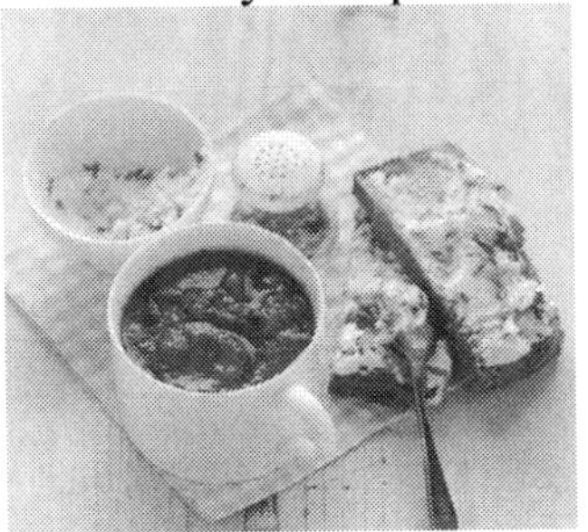

Ingredients:
14 ounces of bag frozen vegetable mix
A sprigs basil, finely chopped
2 tablespoons of garlic, finely chopped
14 ounces of canned tomatoes
1 vegetable stock cube
2 cups of water
4 rye bread slices, toasted
Salt and black pepper to taste

Directions:

1. Heat up a pan at a medium-high temperature. Add half of the vegetable. Mix with garlic. Cook for 5 minutes.
2. Add basil, stock cube, tomatoes, and water. Cook for 5 more minutes.
3. Take off heat. Blend with your kitchen blender. Season with salt and pepper to taste.
4. Heat up the soup again. Add the rest of the vegetables. Cover. Cook for 20 minutes.
5. Pour into the serving bowls. Serve with rye bread.

Enjoy!

Nutritional value: 200 calories, 7 grams of fat, 10 grams of carbs, 6 grams of protein, 13 grams of fiber

Mushroom and Greens Stew

Try this creamy vegetable korma!

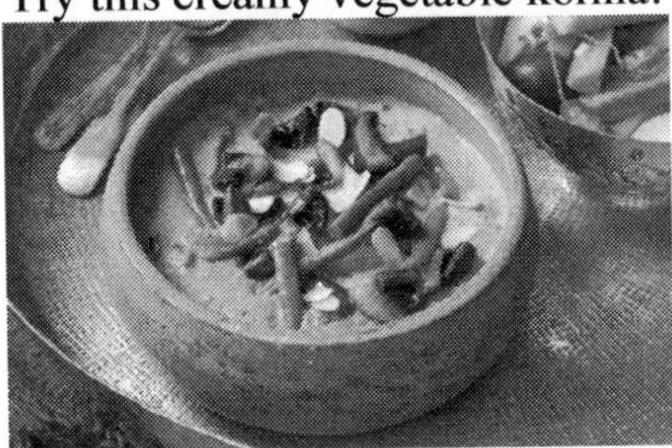

Ingredients:
½ teaspoon of coconut oil
1 garlic clove, chopped
1 red onion, sliced
A small piece of ginger, grated
1 green chili, chopped
½ teaspoon of garam masala
¼ teaspoon of cinnamon
1 teaspoon of cashew nuts
5 ounces of almond milk
1 teaspoon of flaked almonds
6 ounces of mushrooms, sliced
3 ounces of snap peas
1 tablespoon of dried apricots, chopped
Salt and pepper to taste

Directions:

1. Heat up a pan with the oil, at a low heat. Cook onion, chili, ginger, garlic, salt, pepper, garam masala, cinnamon, and cardamom. Cook for 3 minutes.
2. Add almond milk and nuts. Cook for 7 minutes.
3. Pour into a blender. Pulse well. Leave aside.
4. Heat up the same pan at a medium temperature. Cook mushrooms for 2-3 minutes.
5. Add peas, apricots and the sauce you blended earlier. Stir and cook for 8 minutes.
6. Pour into serving bowls. Enjoy.

Nutritional value: 173 calories, 10 grams of fat, 13 grams of carbs, 15 grams of protein, 8 grams of fiber

Healthy Bean Soup

Healthy and delicious soup!

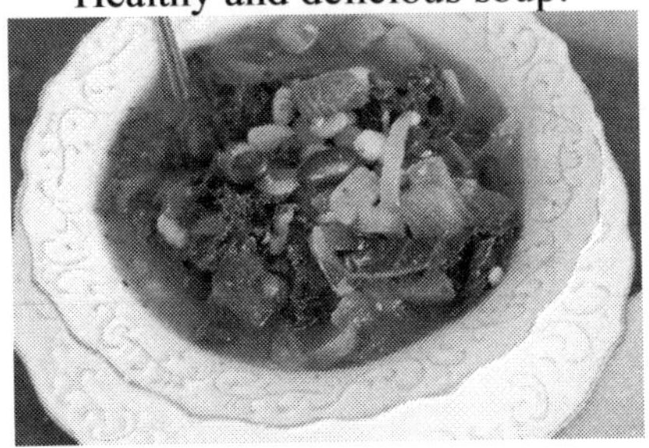

Ingredients:
1 yellow onion, chopped
1 tablespoon of extra-virgin olive oil
6 garlic cloves, crushed
4 cups of vegetable broth
4 cups of fresh chopped kale
2 cups of canned carrots, chopped
2 cups of canned navy beans
3 and ½ cups of chopped tomatoes
2 teaspoons of Italian seasoning
A sprig of chopped parsley
Salt and pepper to taste

Directions:

1. Heat up a large pot with the olive oil, at a medium temperature. Cook the onions and the garlic for 4-5 minutes.
2. Add the kale. Cook for another 10 minutes. Stir constantly.
3. Add the vegetable broth, carrots, beans and tomatoes. Mix well.
4. Bring to a boil. Cook for another 8-9 minutes.
5. Add the Italian seasoning, chopped parsley, and salt and pepper to taste.
6. Boil for another 2-3 minutes. Serve!

Enjoy!

Nutritional value: 192 calories, 1 grams of fat, 30 grams of carbs, 12 grams of fiber, 10 grams of protein

Tasty Lunch Cucumber Salad

Tasty salad with finely chopped ingredients!

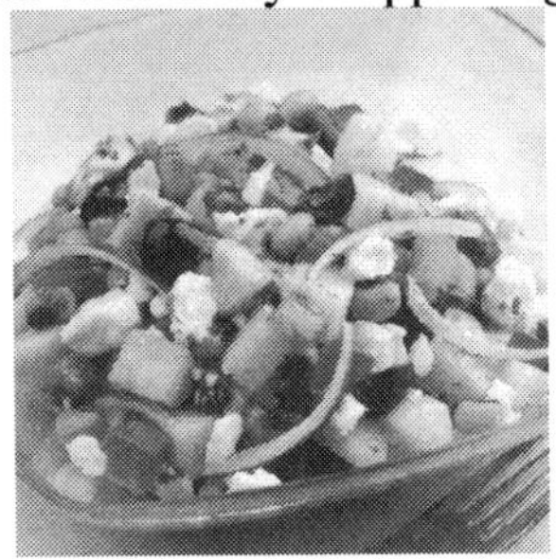

Ingredients:
3 tablespoons of extra-virgin olive oil
2 tablespoons of lemon juice
Salt and black pepper to taste
2 teaspoons of chopped oregano
4 cups of cucumbers, cubed
14 ounces of canned black-eyed peas, drained
½ cup of goat cheese, crumbled
½ cup of red onion, finely chopped
2 tablespoons of black olives, pitted and chopped
½ cup of red bell pepper, chopped

Directions:

1. Mix olive oil with salt, pepper, oregano and lemon juice. Stir. Pour into a bowl. Leave aside for now.
2. Put cucumber, peas, bell pepper, onion, cheese and olives in a bowl. Stir.
3. Add salad dressing. Toss to coat. Serve cold!

Enjoy!

Nutritional value: 89 calories, 1 grams of fat, 3 grams of carbs, 5 grams of protein, 3 grams of fibers

Delicious Lettuce and Fennel Salad

The best taste, the best colors

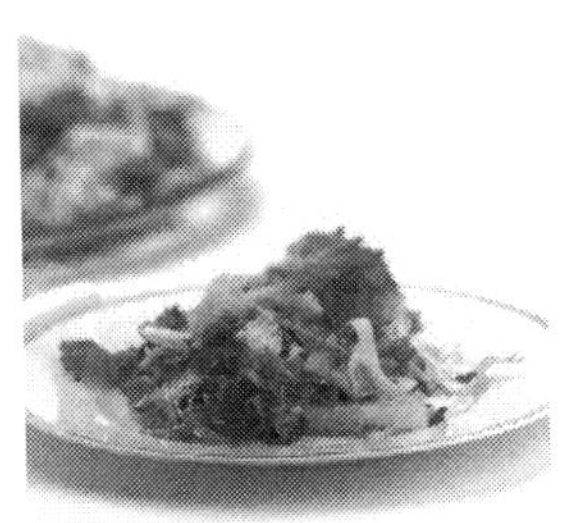

Ingredients:
1 tablespoon of red wine vinegar
1 cups of olive oil
1 teaspoon of mustard
1 tablespoon of lemon juice
2 garlic cloves, finely chopped
½ cup of Kalamata olives, chopped
1 tablespoon of parsley, chopped
10 cups of mixed lettuces, such as chicory, radicchio, and leaf lettuce
2 endive heads, sliced
3 medium navel oranges, peeled and cut lengthwise
2 bulbs fennel, thinly sliced
Salt and black pepper to taste

Directions:

1. In a bowl, mix vinegar with lemon juice, garlic, salt, pepper, and mustard. Stir well. Leave aside.
2. Add oil. Stir again.
3. Add olives and parsley. Stir. Leave aside.
4. In a large salad bowl, combine mixed lettuces with fennel, endive, and oranges.
5. Drizzle dressing on top. Toss to coat. Serve!

Enjoy!

Nutritional value: 75 calories, 1 grams of fat, 2 grams of carbs, 5 grams of protein, 3 grams of fibers

Tasty Barley Soup

Barley soup with many spices to add great flavor!

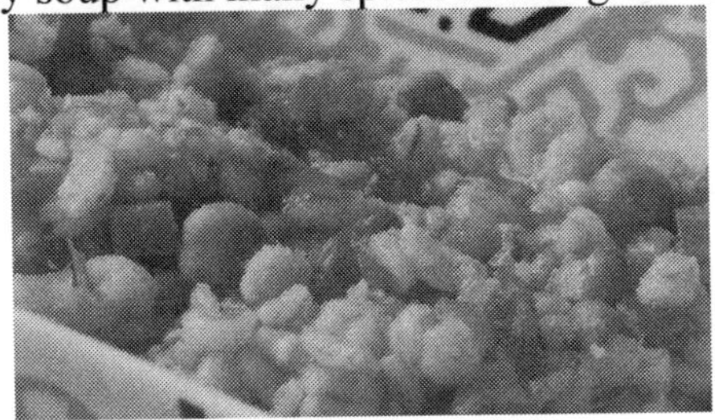

Ingredients:
2 quarts of vegetable broth
1 cup of uncooked barley
2 celery stalks, chopped
2 carrots, chopped
14 ounces of canned tomatoes (and juice), chopped
1 zucchini, chopped
3 bay leaves
15 ounces of canned garbanzo beans, drained
1 yellow onion, chopped
1 teaspoon of parsley, dried
1 teaspoon of garlic powder
1 teaspoon of curry powder
1 teaspoon of Worcestershire sauce
1 teaspoon of paprika
Salt and black pepper to taste

Directions:

1. Pour vegetable broth in a pot. Add carrots, barley, tomatoes, zucchini, tomatoes, beans, celery, onion and bay leaves.
2. Season with salt, pepper, parsley, garlic powder, curry powder, paprika, and Worcestershire sauce. Bring to a boil on the stove at a medium-low temperature. Cook for 90 minutes.
3. Discard bay leaves. Pour into the serving bowls. Serve!

Enjoy!

Nutritional value: 140 calories, 3 grams of fat, 3 grams of carbs, 7 grams of protein, 6 grams of fibers

Carrot and Coriander Soup

This soup has such a creamy taste!

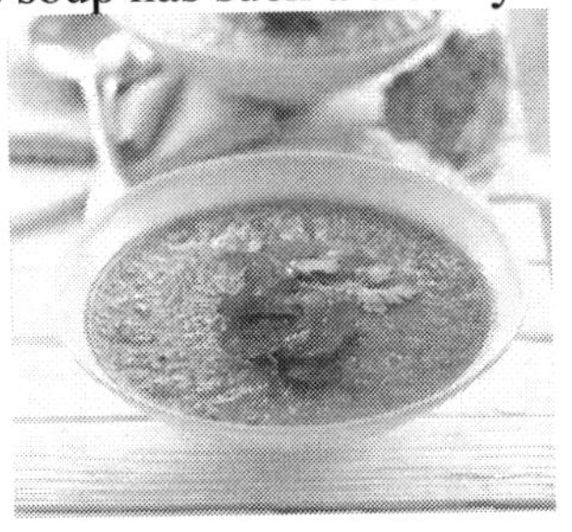

Ingredients:
2 tablespoons of extra-virgin olive oil
1 yellow onion, chopped
2 large garlic cloves, finely chopped
1 pound of carrots, peeled and chopped
1/ teaspoon of coriander
¼ teaspoon of ground chili
2 cups of vegetable stock
A spring of fresh coriander, finely chopped
Salt and black pepper to taste

Directions:

1. Heat up a large pot with the oil over the stove, at a medium-high temperature. Cook the onion for 2-3 minutes. Stir constantly.
2. Add garlic. Stir and cook for 3 more minutes.
3. Add carrots. Cook for 4 minutes.
4. Add chili, coriander, salt, pepper and vegetable broth. Stir. Cover. Reduce heat. Cook for 20 minutes.
5. Remove pot from heat. Add fresh coriander. Blend using your kitchen blender.
6. Pour into the serving bowls while it's still hot. Serve right away!

Enjoy!

Nutritional value: 130 calories, 2 grams of fat, 4 grams of carbs, 4 grams of fiber, 7 grams of protein

Spicy Beans with Tasty Polenta

You won't feel full after eating this one!

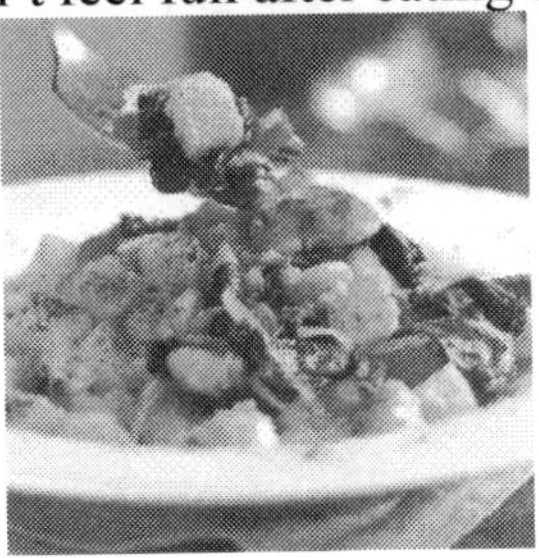

Ingredients:
4 teaspoons of extra-virgin olive oil
16 ounces of plain polenta cut into small cubes
1 garlic clove crushed
½ teaspoon of smoked paprika
¾ cup of vegetable broth
1 yellow onion, thinly sliced
1 red bell pepper, chopped
15 ounces of canned butter beans, drained
4 cups of baby spinach
½ cup of goat cheese, shredded
2 teaspoons of sherry vinegar

Directions:

1. Heat up a pan with 2 teaspoons of oil, at a medium-high temperature. Add polenta in a single layer. Cook for 8 minutes. Stir gently occasionally. Transfer onto a plate.
2. Reduce heat to medium. Add the rest of the oil to the pan and garlic. Cook for 30 seconds. Stir occasionally.
3. Add onion, paprika and bell pepper. Cook for 6 minutes.
4. Add beans, spinach and broth. Cook for 3 minutes more.
5. Remove from heat. Add cheese and vinegar. Transfer onto serving platters. Top with vegetable mix.

Enjoy!

Nutritional value: 160 calories, 5 grams of fat, 7 grams of carbs, 5 grams of fiber, 10 grams of protein

Turkish Style Vegetarian Salad

As colorful as it is perfect!

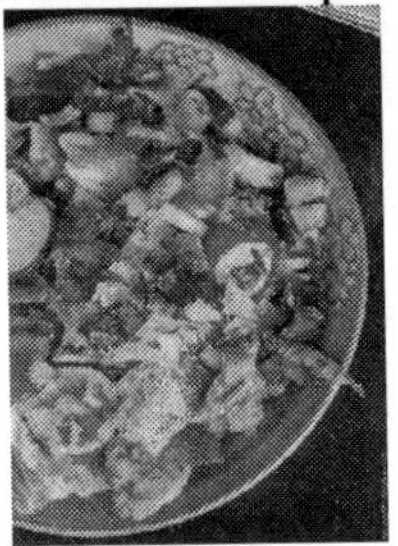

Ingredients:
3 tablespoons of olive oil
2 loaves pita bread
1 cucumber, cubed
5 tomatoes, roughly chopped
1 lettuce heart, chopped
½ teaspoon of sumac
1 cup of parsley, finely chopped
5 green peppers, chopped
5 radishes, thinly sliced
For the salad dressing:
1/3 cup of olive oil
Juice from 1½ limes
½ teaspoon of cinnamon
1 teaspoon of sumac
¼ teaspoon of allspice
Salt and black pepper to taste

Directions:

1. Toast pita bread. Arrange on a plate. Leave aside for now.
2. Heat up a pan with 3 tablespoons of olive oil, at a medium temperature. Break pita and add it to the pan. Brown for 2 minutes. Add salt, pepper and ½ teaspoon of sumac.
3. Transfer pita onto paper towels. Drain. Leave aside for now.
4. In a bowl, mix lettuce with onion, cucumber, tomatoes, parsley and radishes. Leave aside as well.
5. In another bowl, mix 1/3 cup of olive oil with lime juice, salt, pepper, 1 teaspoon of sumac, cinnamon, and allspice. Stir.
6. Mix salad with this dressing. Toss to coat. Top with toasted pita.

Enjoy!

Nutritional value: 120 calories, 0 grams of fat, 1 grams of carbs, 6 grams of protein, 5 grams of fibers

Tofu and Eggplant Packages

This is another super-delicious dish for you to try as soon as possible!

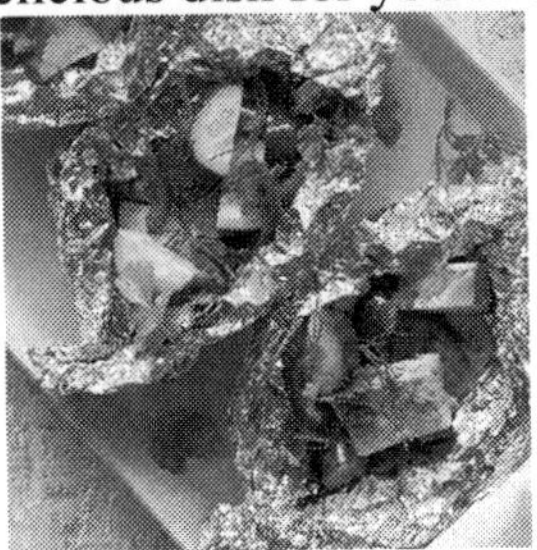

Ingredients:
20 ounces of firm tofu, cut into 16 pieces
12 ounces of eggplant, cut into medium-sized chunks
7 tablespoons of olive oil
2 tablespoons of garlic, crushed
2 tablespoons of ginger, grated
¼ cup of soy sauce
1 cup of dill, roughly chopped
2 green onions, finely chopped
1 cucumber, cut into chunks
2 tablespoons of lime juice
1 cup of cilantro, roughly chopped
1 red jalapeno pepper, sliced
Sea salt and black pepper to taste

Directions:

1. Place tofu in a zip-top bag. Add eggplant pieces, garlic, ginger, soy sauce, green onions, salt, pepper and 5 tablespoons of oil. Seal. Shake well. Leave aside for now.
2. Heat up your kitchen grill. Divide the tofu mix onto 4 pieces of high-quality tin foil. Wrap them. Place on grill. Cook for 10 minutes. Turn them once. Transfer to a platter. Unwrap. Leave aside to cool down for 1-2 minutes.
3. In a bowl, mix cucumber with cilantro, jalapeno, dill, lime juice, 2 tablespoons of oil, and some salt and pepper. Stir well.
4. Serve tofu and eggplant packages with the cucumber salad on the side.

Enjoy!

Nutritional value: 180 calories, 10 grams of fat, 20 grams of carbs, 0 grams of fiber, 5 grams of protein

Avocado and Goat Cheese Quesadilla

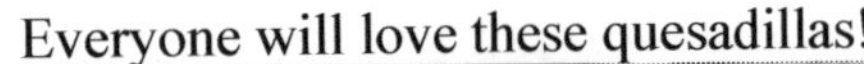
Everyone will love these quesadillas!

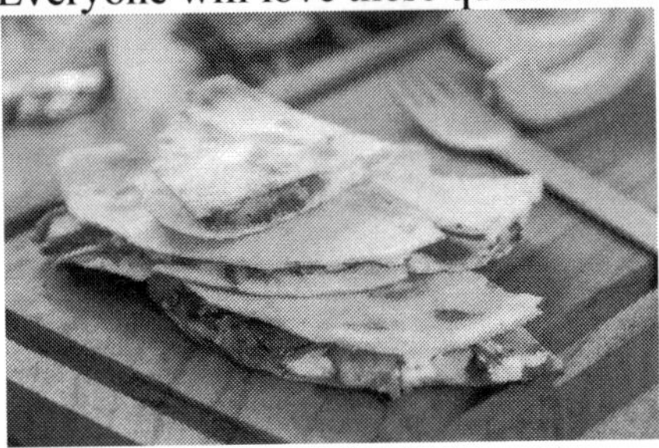

Ingredients:
4 whole wheat tortillas
1 ripe avocado
8 tablespoons of crumbled goat cheese
A pinch of salt and black pepper
1 tablespoon of lemon juice
A sprigs cilantro, roughly chopped
1 teaspoon of extra-virgin olive oil

Directions:

1. In a bowl, mix avocado with lemon juice. Stir.
2. Divide avocado pieces and goat cheese between two tortillas.
3. Sprinkle cilantro, a pinch of salt, and pepper. Brush with the oil.
4. Heat up a grill pan at a medium-high temperature. Grill each tortilla side for about 3 minutes.
5. Transfer to a platter. Cut into quarters. Serve with your favorite tortilla dressing.

Enjoy your lunch!

Nutritional value: 400 calories, 20 grams of fat, 28 grams of carbs, 13 grams of fiber, 18 grams of protein

Amazing Mexican Rice

This Mexican rice may be the best lunch you'll ever have!

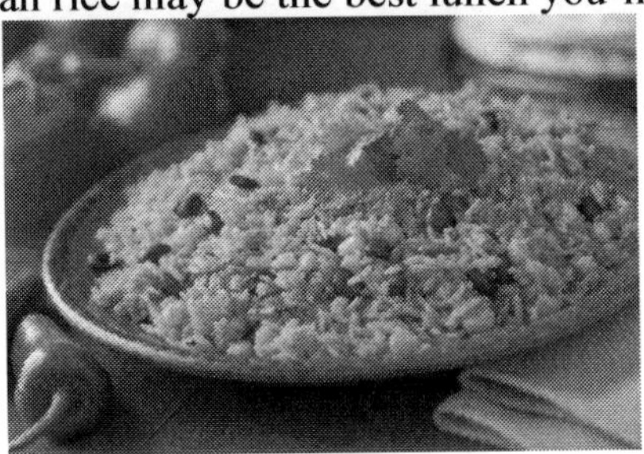

Ingredients:
1 tablespoon of extra-virgin olive oil
1 yellow onion, finely chopped
2 celery stalks, finely chopped
2 garlic cloves, finely chopped
2 cups of brown rice
1½ cup of canned black beans, rinsed and drained
4 cups of water
2 cups of corn kernels
Salt and black pepper to taste

Directions:

1. Heat up a saucepan with the olive oil, at a medium-high temperature. Cook celery and onion for 8 minutes. Stir constantly.
2. Add corn, beans and garlic. Stir and sauté them for about 5 minutes.
3. Add the rice, water, and salt and pepper to taste. Stir. Cover. Reduce heat. Cook for 45 minutes.
4. Take rice off heat. Transfer onto plates. Serve right away!

Enjoy!

Nutritional value: 199 calories, 8 grams of fat, 28 grams of carbs, 3 grams of protein, 2 grams of fiber

Vegetarian Chili with Peppers

This is a tasteful vegetarian dish! Try it!

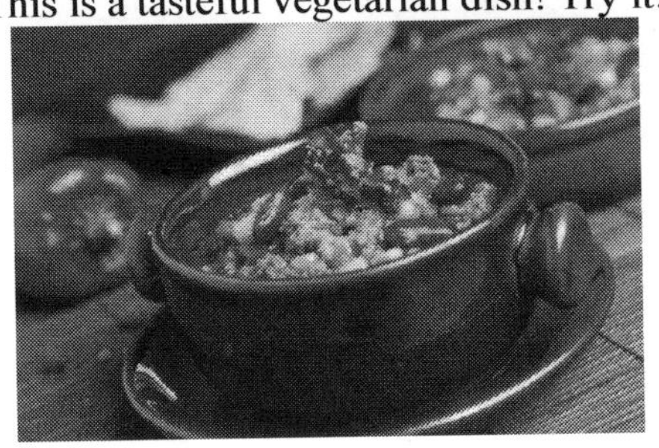

Ingredients:
2 tablespoons of extra-virgin olive oil
1 yellow onion, finely chopped
1 celery rib, finely chopped
2 garlic cloves, minced
1 pound of frozen green, yellow and red bell peppers
2½ cups of canned black beans, rinsed and drained
2 teaspoons of cumin
1 teaspoon of oregano
2 tablespoons of orange juice
1 tablespoon of lemon juice
2 cups of canned tomatoes and green chilies, chopped
½ teaspoon of hot sauce
2 tablespoons of cilantro, finely chopped
Salt and black pepper to taste

Directions:

1. Heat up a large pot with the oil, at a medium-high temperature. Cook celery, onion, bell peppers mix and garlic for 5 minutes.
2. Add cumin and oregano. Stir and cook for 2 more minutes.
3. Add the beans, tomatoes, chilies, orange and lemon juice, and hot sauce. Bring to a boil. Cover. Reduce heat. Boil for about 25 minutes.
4. Season with salt and pepper to taste. Add cilantro at the end. Stir. Transfer onto plates. Serve right away.

Enjoy!

Nutritional value: 260, 2 grams of fat, 60 grams of carbs, 14 grams of fiber, 19 grams of protein

Vegetarian Burritos

You wouldn't expect a vegetarian dish to taste so good!

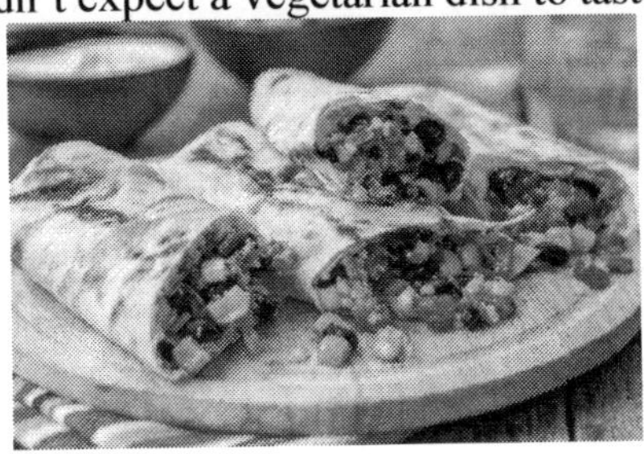

Ingredients:
1 tablespoon of extra-virgin olive oil
1 yellow onion, finely chopped
2 small garlic cloves, minced
2 green bell peppers, finely chopped
2 red bell peppers, finely chopped
½ cup of canned corn, drained and rinsed
2 cups of canned black beans, drained and rinsed
2 tablespoons of cilantro, finely chopped
1 teaspoon of cumin
2 tablespoons of lime juice
1½ teaspoon of chili powder
10 whole wheat tortillas
2 cups of pre-cooked quinoa
Salt and black pepper to taste

Directions:

1. Heat up a saucepan with the oil, at a medium-high temperature. Sauté the onion for 4-5 minutes.
2. Add garlic. Stir and cook for 1 minute more.
3. Add beans, corn, red and green peppers, cilantro, chili powder, and cumin. Stir well and cook for 5 minutes.
4. Add lime juice, salt and pepper to taste. Take off heat.
5. Scoop quinoa onto each tortilla. Add beans and corn mixture roll. Place in a heated pan. Warm them up for 2-3 minutes.
6. Transfer to plates. Serve!

Enjoy!

Nutritional value: 320, 18 grams of fat, 18 grams of carbs, 12 grams of fiber, 24 grams of protein

Vegetarian Salad Boats

A delicious and nutritious vegetarian dish!

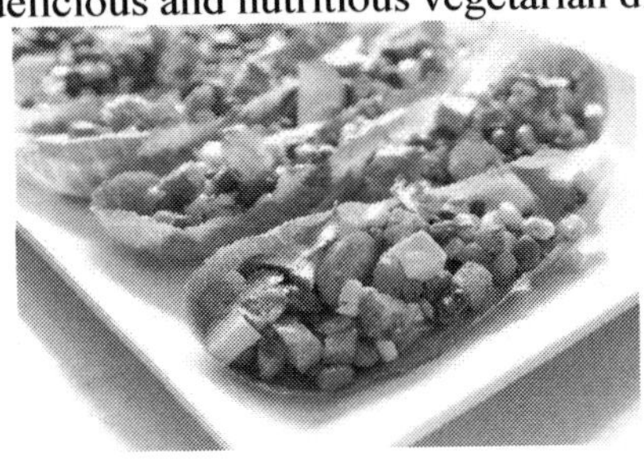

Ingredients:
1 sprig of salad leaves, rinsed
4 tablespoons of extra-virgin olive oil
1 teaspoon of chili powder
1 teaspoon of cumin
1½ cup of canned black beans, drained and rinsed
1½ cup of canned corn, drained and rinsed
1 sweet potato, finely chopped
Juice from 1 lime
10 cherry tomatoes, halved
½ cup of cilantro, finely chopped
1 avocado ripened
4 radishes thinly sliced
Salt and black pepper to taste

Directions:

1. Heat up a pan with half of the oil, at a medium-high temperature. Cook the potatoes for 2-3 minutes.
2. Add salt, pepper, cumin and chili powder. Stir. Cook for 10 minutes. Take off heat. Leave aside.
3. In a bowl, mix the rest of the oil with the lime juice, salt, pepper, and cilantro.
4. In a salad bowl, mix corn, beans, tomatoes, radishes and sweet potatoes.
5. Add the cilantro dressing you prepared earlier. Toss to coat.
6. Fill each lettuce leaf with this mix. Top with avocado. Serve!

Enjoy!

Nutritional value: 100 calories, 2 grams of fat, 16 grams of carbs, 2 grams of fiber, 5 grams of protein

Mexican Style Quinoa Burgers

A Mexican style recipe that will suit all tastes!

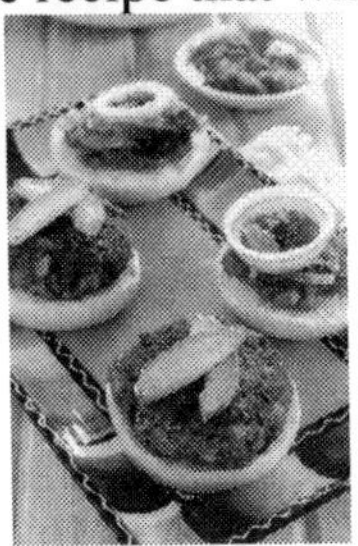

Ingredients:
Cooking spray
1 green bell pepper, finely chopped
4 garlic cloves, finely chopped
1 yellow onion, finely chopped
1½ cups of canned black beans, drained and rinsed
1½ cups of pre-cooked quinoa
½ cup of cheddar cheese, crumbled
2 tablespoons of taco seasoning
1 teaspoon of paprika
1 cup of breadcrumbs
2 tablespoons of flaxseeds, soaked and mixed with 6 tablespoons of warm water
Coconut oil for frying
2 tablespoons of salsa
Avocado slices and lettuce leaves for serving

Directions:

1. Spray some cooking spray in a pan. Heat up at a medium-high temperature. Cook onion and pepper for 10 minutes. Stir occasionally.
2. Add garlic. Stir. Cook for 2 minutes. Remove from heat. Transfer into a bowl. Leave aside for now.
3. Meanwhile, put half of the quinoa and half of the beans in your blender. Pulse a few times.
4. Add this mix to onions. Stir.
5. Add flaxseeds, cheese, bread crumbs, taco seasoning, paprika and the rest of the quinoa and the beans. Stir. Leave aside for 5 minutes. Shape your burgers using your hands and arrange them on a working surface.
6. Heat up a pan with the coconut oil, at a medium-high temperature. Add quinoa burgers and fry them for a few minutes. Flip them only once.
7. Place them on sliced buns. Serve with lettuce leaves and avocado slices.
8. Serve in sliced buns with salsa, avocado slices and lettuce leaves.

Enjoy!

Nutritional value: 190 calories, 13 grams of fat, 20 grams of carbs, 3 grams of fiber, 5 grams of protein

Gourmet Porridge with Cilantro

A unique porridge to try!

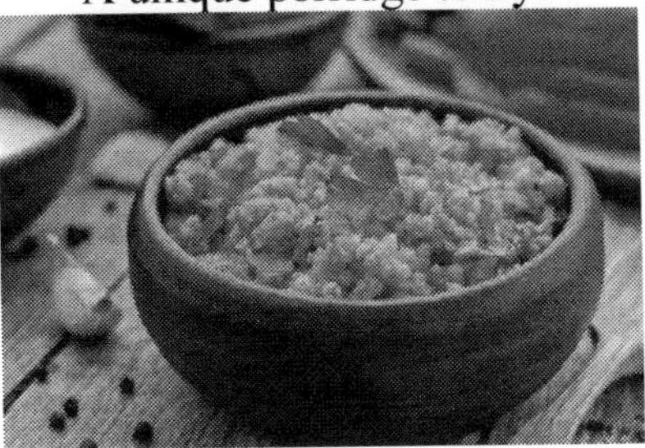

Ingredients:
4 tablespoons of extra-virgin olive oil
1 cup of millet, rinsed
2 small bunches green onions, finely chopped
2 tomatoes, finely chopped
½ cup of cilantro, finely chopped
5 drops Tabasco sauce
6 cups of cold water
½ cup of lemon juice
Salt and black pepper to taste

Directions:

1. Heat up a pan with 2 tablespoons of olive oil, at a medium-high temperature. Cook millet for 4 minutes.
2. Add water. Bring to a boil. Cover. Boil for 20 minutes.
3. Drain. Rinse. Drain again. Transfer millet into a bowl.
4. Add tomatoes, onions, lemon juice, cilantro, hot sauce, salt, pepper and the rest of the oil.
5. Toss to coat. Serve right away!

Enjoy!

Nutritional value: 120 calories, 6 grams of fat, 4 grams of carbs, 2 grams of fiber, 14 grams of protein

Lunch Omelet Wrap

You've never tasted something like this before!

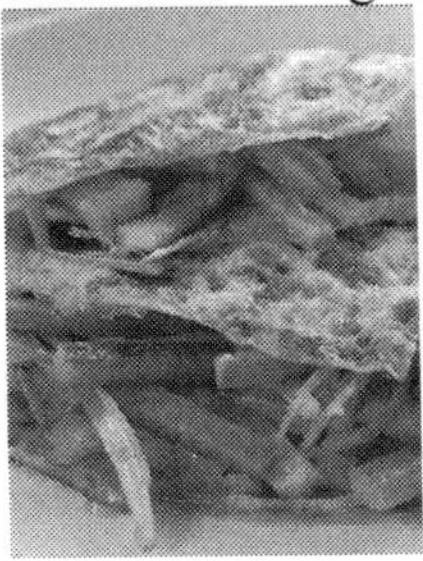

Ingredients:
4 tablespoons of coconut milk
4 eggs
2 teaspoons of sesame oil
2 teaspoons of soy sauce
1 carrot, thinly sliced
1 courgette, cut into thin strips
2 spring onions, cut into strips
1½ tablespoons of chili sauce
Salt and black pepper to taste

Directions:

1. Whisk eggs in a bowl and season them with salt and pepper.
2. Heat up a pan with 1 tablespoon of olive oil, at a medium-high temperature. Pour half of the eggs. Spread mix in the pan evenly. Cook omelet for 2 minutes. Transfer onto a plate. Leave aside for now.
3. Pour the rest of the egg mix into the same pan. Cook this omelet for 2 minutes. Transfer to the same plate.
4. Heat up the rest of the oil in the same pan. Add carrot slices, courgette and spring onion strips. Cook for 3 minutes. Stir constantly.
5. Add soy sauce, salt and pepper. Cook for 1 more minute. Take off heat.
6. Drizzle chili sauce over omelet. Add vegetable mix on top. Fold and serve!

Enjoy!

Nutritional value: 265 calories, 14 grams of fats, grams of proteins 13, 3 grams of fibers

Gourmet Lunch Salad

This special lunch salad is what you need!

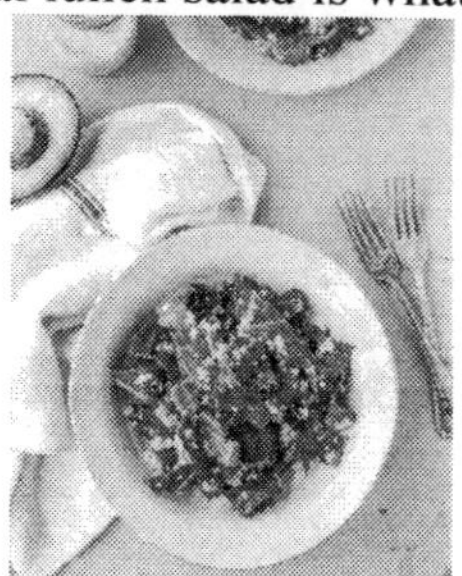

Ingredients:
1 cup of pre-cooked cooked quinoa
1 avocado, roughly chopped
1 medium-sized bunch of collard greens, thinly chopped
1 sprigs of strawberries, sliced
4 tablespoons of chopped walnuts
2 tablespoons of white wine vinegar
1 teaspoon of white miso
4 tablespoons of tahini
4 tablespoons of cold water
1 tablespoon of maple syrup

Directions:

1. Mix tahini with maple syrup, water, vinegar and miso in your blender. Pulse a few times. Transfer into a bowl. Leave aside.
2. In a salad bowl, mix collard green leaves with half of the salad dressing. Toss to coat.
3. Add avocado, walnuts, quinoa and strawberries. Toss again
4. Add the rest of the dressing on top. Serve!

Enjoy!

Nutritional value: 230 calories, grams of fats 13, grams of proteins 6, grams of fibers 4

Grain Salad with Avocado Dressing

This delicious salad is just what you need to continue the day!

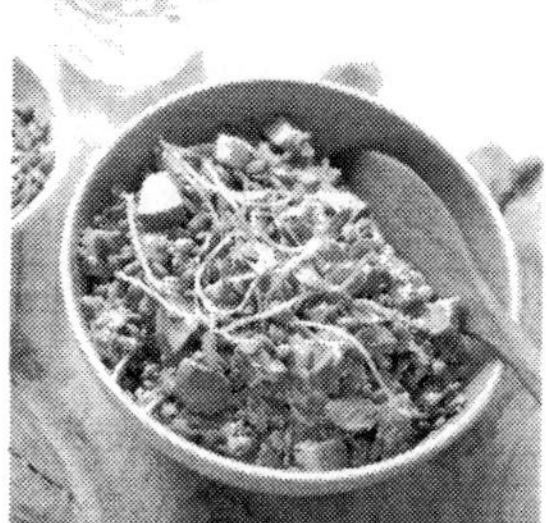

Ingredients:
10 tablespoons of roasted pepitas
3 cups of water
1 sprigs cilantro, finely chopped
4 tablespoons of parsley, finely chopped
1½ cups of raw einkorn
1 cup of radish sprouts
2 avocados, roughly chopped
2 mangos, chopped
3 tablespoons of extra-virgin olive oil
4 tablespoons of coconut yogurt
1 teaspoons of sherry vinegar
2 tablespoons of lemon juice
Salt and black pepper to taste

Directions:

1. Mix olive oil with avocados, salt, pepper, lemon juice and vinegar.
2. Put this in your blender. Pulse a few times.
3. Add yogurt. Pulse again. Transfer into a bowl. Leave aside for now.
4. Heat up a large pot with water, at a medium-high temperature. Add einkorn. Bring to a boil. Reduce heat. Simmer for about 30 minutes.
5. Drain einkorn. Transfer into a bowl. Leave aside.
6. In a salad bowl, mix pepitas with einkorn, parsley, cilantro, radish sprouts, mango, and salt and pepper to taste.
7. Add salad dressing. Toss to coat. Serve!

Enjoy!

Nutritional value: 338 calories, grams of fats 22, 8 grams of proteins, 3 grams of fibers

Beans, Caramelized Onions, and Almonds

This is truly a wonderful lunch recipe!

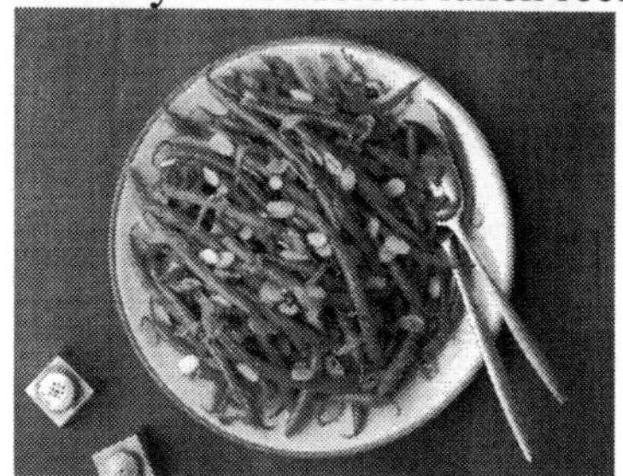

Ingredients:
5 tablespoons of extra-virgin olive oil
3 pounds of green beans, halved and boiled in salted water for 5 minutes
8 tablespoons of almonds, sliced
Salt and black pepper to taste
2 yellow onions, finely chopped
2 and ½ tablespoons of thyme, finely chopped

Directions:

1. Heat up a large pan at a medium-high temperature. Cook the beans for 5 minutes. Take off heat. Transfer into a bowl. Leave aside.
2. Toast almonds in the same pan for 3 minutes. Take off heat. Transfer into the same bowl as the beans. Leave aside.
3. Return the pan to stove. Add olive oil. Put heat on medium. Cook the onions with salt and pepper for about 20 minutes. Stir occasionally.
4. Add thyme. Cook for 5 minutes.
5. Add beans and almonds. Season to taste. Cook for another 4 minutes. Transfer onto serving plates!

Nutritional value: 170 calories, 15 grams of fats, 4 grams of proteins, 3 grams of fibers

Delicious Tomato and Peach Salad

The best way to end your day!

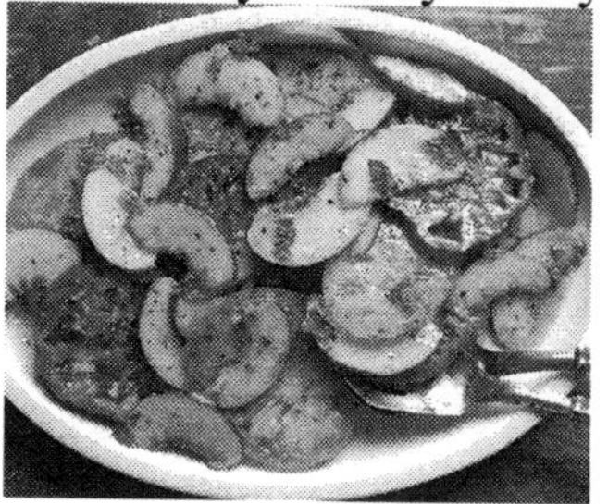

Ingredients:
3 cups of marinated peaches, drained and sliced
½ bunch mint, finely chopped
4 plum tomatoes, sliced
1 teaspoon of mustard
1 tablespoon of sherry and rosemary vinegar
Salt and black pepper to taste

Directions:

1. In a bowl, mix vinegar with mustard, salt, and pepper. Stir. Leave aside.
2. Put tomato slices on separate serving plates. Add peaches and half of the vinaigrette.
3. Add mint. Toss to coat. Serve with the rest of the vinaigrette on top.

Enjoy!

Nutritional value: 70 calories, 2 grams of fats, 4 grams of proteins, 2 grams of fibers

Wow Salad

This salad will make you say wow!

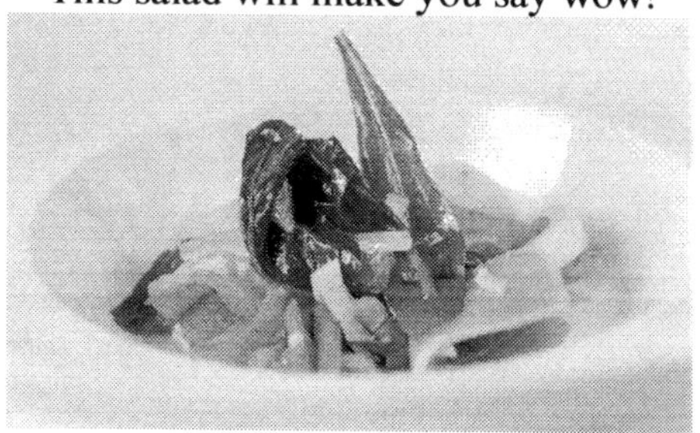

Ingredients:
1 tablespoon of extra-virgin olive oil
7 ounces of pasta
1 zucchini, roughly sliced
1 fennel, roughly chopped
½ lettuce leaves, roughly chopped
2 beets, roughly chopped
1 small bunch green asparagus, halved
2 zucchini flowers, chopped
Juice from 1 lemon
1 handful of your favorite fresh herbs, roughly chopped
Salt and black pepper to taste

Directions:

1. Cook pasta. Drain. Transfer to a bowl. Leave aside for now.
2. Put zucchini, asparagus, fennel and beets in a pot. Cover with water. Add a pinch of salt. Boil for 3-4 minutes in salted water. Drain. Transfer to a salad bowl.
3. Add zucchini flowers, salad leaves, pasta, salt, pepper, fresh herbs, lemon juice and olive oil. Toss to coat. Serve!

Enjoy!

Nutritional value: 340 calories, 4 grams of fats 4, 10 grams of proteins, 7 grams of carbs, 2 grams of fibers

Fancy Zucchini Dish

This will soon become your favorite dinner recipe!

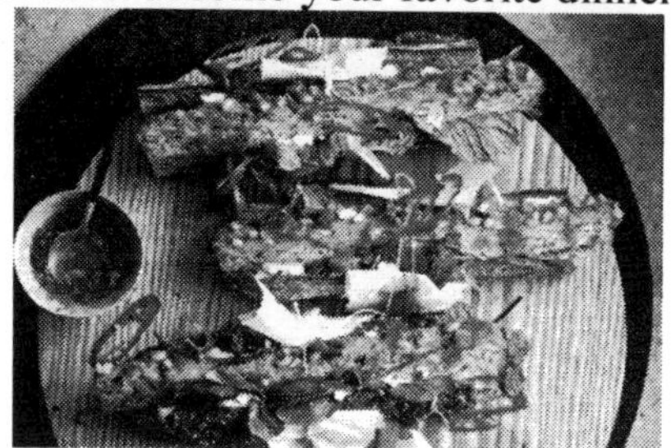

Ingredients:
2 tablespoons of extra-virgin olive oil
4 zucchinis, thinly sliced
2 garlic cloves, thinly sliced
1 yellow onion, finely chopped
1 carrots, finely sliced
Zest from 1 lemon
5 eggs
1 teaspoon of chili flakes
1 baguette, sliced lengthways
2 tablespoons of pine nuts, finely chopped
4 tablespoons of mint, finely chopped
2 tablespoons of coriander, chopped
2 tablespoons of almond flour
Salt and black pepper to taste
A small bunch mixed salad leaves, cut into medium chunks
1 cup of cheddar cheese, grated

Directions:

1. Mix zucchini slices with carrot, salt, and pepper. Stir. Leave aside for 5 minutes. Drain liquid. Place in a bowl.
2. Heat up a pan with the oil, at a medium-high temperature. Cook the onion for 3 minutes.
3. Add lemon zest, garlic and chili. Cook for 1 minute. Take off heat. Leave aside.
4. In a bowl, whisk eggs with almond flour.
5. Add carrots, zucchinis, pine nuts, onion, cheese, and coriander. Stir well.
6. Pour egg mix into an oven-proof dish. Put food in the oven. Bake at 200 degrees F for 25 minutes.
7. Take omelet out of the oven. Leave it to cool down for a few minutes. Cut into strips.
8. Fill the baguette with salad leaves, mint leaves and the omelet you prepared earlier.

Enjoy!

Nutritional value: 140 calories, 7 grams of fats, 7 grams of proteins, 1 gram of fibers

Artichoke Pizza

Do you want to eat something really good for dinner? Try this pizza!

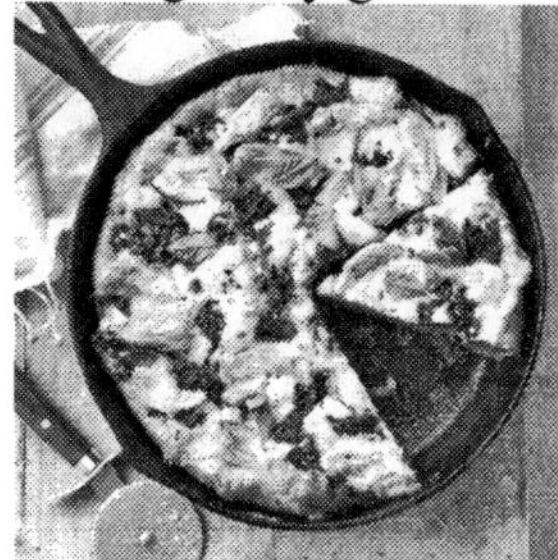

Ingredients:
1 tablespoon of extra-virgin olive oil
3 garlic cloves, finely chopped
5 ounces of baby spinach, chopped
1½ ounces of parmesan cheese, grated
½ cup of ricotta cheese
¼ teaspoon of red pepper flakes
1 tablespoon of lemon juice
Salt and black pepper to taste
1 pound vegetarian pizza dough
1½ tablespoons of cornmeal
6 ounces of fontina cheese, grated
14 ounces of canned artichoke hearts, drained
Some basil leaves, roughly chopped for serving

Directions:

1. Heat up a pan with the oil, at a medium temperature. Add garlic and spinach. Cook for 4 minutes while stirring gently. Drain. Transfer to a plate.
2. In a bowl, mix ricotta with lemon juice, parmesan cheese, red pepper flakes, salt, and pepper. Stir well.
3. Sprinkle the pan where you cooked the spinach with cornmeal. Press dough into the skillet. Spread ricotta mix, artichokes, spinach mix and fontina.
4. Put food in the oven at 450 degrees F. Bake for 24 minutes.
5. Take out of the oven. Leave to cool down for 5 minutes. Cut. Sprinkle basil on top. Serve!

Enjoy!

Nutritional value: 676 calories, 32 grams of fat, 76 grams of carbs, 5 grams of fiber, 32 grams of protein

Tofu Sandwiches

Is there a better way to end the day than eating these?

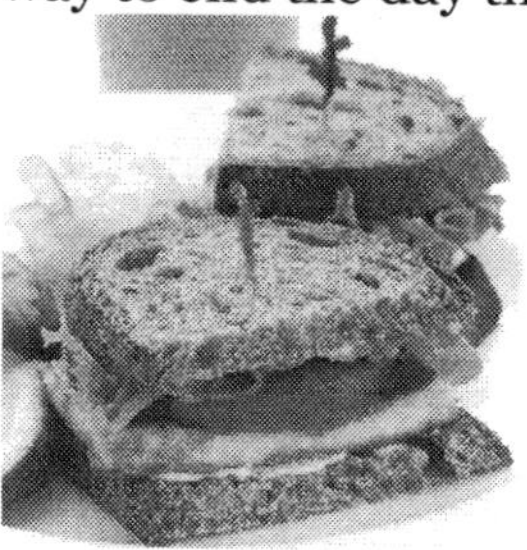

Ingredients:
1 tablespoon of soy sauce
1 teaspoon of adobo sauce
1 tablespoon of Dijon mustard
14 ounces of extra firm tofu, drained and rinsed
8 slices whole wheat bread, toasted
4 lettuce leaves
2 tomatoes, sliced

Directions:

1. In a bowl, mix mustard with ½ a teaspoon of adobo sauce and soy sauce. Stir well.
2. Pat dry tofu slices with paper towels. Arrange them on a baking sheet sprayed with some oil.
3. Spread half of the mustard mix on tofu slices. Flip them. Spread the rest of the mix.
4. Put food in the oven at 475 degrees F. Bake for 20 minutes.
5. Spread the rest of the adobo sauce on 4 toasted slices. Take tofu out of the oven. Divide on bread. Add lettuce and tomato slices. Top with the other 4 slices of bread.

Enjoy!

Nutritional value: 200 calories, 8 grams of fat, 32 grams of carbs, 8 grams of protein, 2 grams of fiber

Cucumber and Watermelon Salad

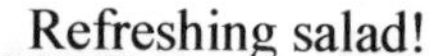

Refreshing salad!

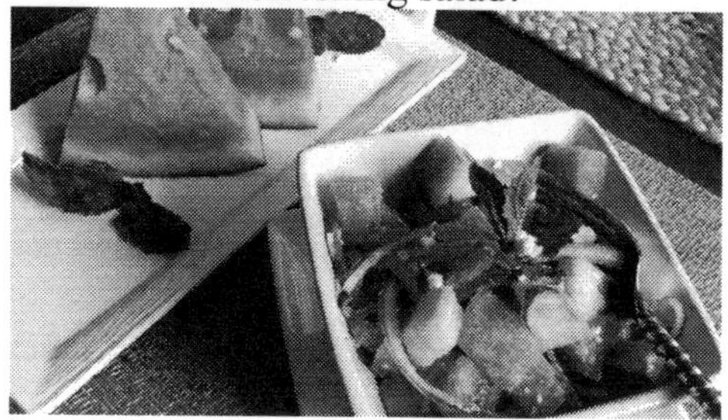

Ingredients:
3 cucumbers, roughly chopped
2 tablespoons of extra-virgin olive oil
1 red onion, sliced
1 small watermelon, cubed
1 cup of favorite cheese, shredded
2 tablespoons of lime juice
½ cup of mint, thinly chopped
Black pepper to taste

Directions:

1. In a bowl, mix onion with lime juice. Toss to coat. Leave aside for a few minutes
2. Add oil. Stir gently.
3. In another bowl, mix watermelon with cucumbers and cheese. Sprinkle some black pepper on top.
4. Add pickled onion. Stir gently. Serve with chopped mint on top.

Enjoy!

Nutritional value: 160 calories, 14 grams of fat, 13 grams of carbs, 3 grams of fiber, 4 grams of protein

Fresh Tomato Salad

A light dinner!

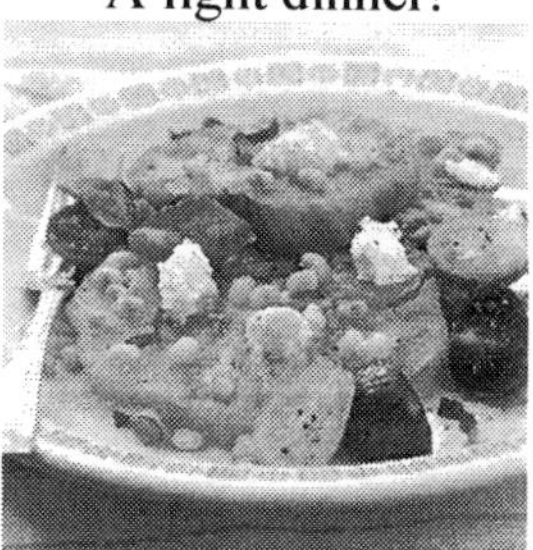

Ingredients:
1 cup of fresh lady peas
2 pounds of plum tomatoes, sliced
4 ounces of goat cheese, crumbled
Salt and black pepper to taste
For the basil dressing:
1/3 cup of canola oil
1 teaspoon of lemon zest
¼ cup of fresh lemon juice
1 tablespoon of Dijon mustard
1 medium bunch basil, finely chopped
Salt to taste
½ teaspoon of ground red pepper

Directions:

1. Mix canola oil with mustard, basil, lemon zest, salt, red pepper and lemon juice. Put everything in your food processor. Pulse a few times.
2. Transfer this mix into a bowl. Leave aside.
3. Heat up a pan with some water, at a medium temperature. Cook peas for 10 minutes.
4. Drain peas. Put in a bowl. Mix them with half of the basil dressing.
5. Put tomato slices on plates. On top, add peas, goat cheese, salt, black pepper and more basil dressing.
6. Toss to coat. Serve!

Enjoy!

Nutritional value: 86 calories, 3 grams of fat, 9 grams of carbs, 2 grams of fiber, 5 grams of protein

Okra and Potato Dish

It's easy to make and so tasty!

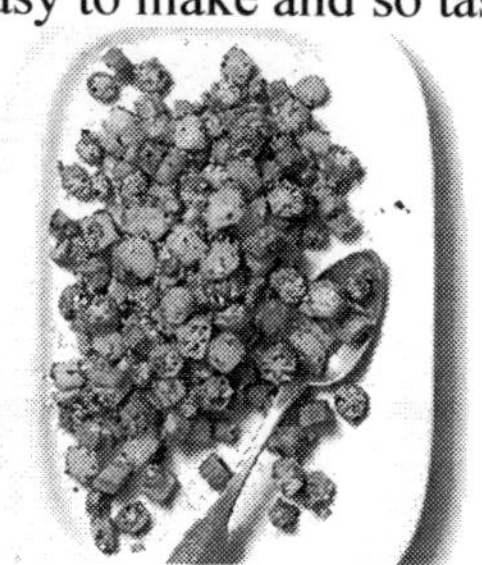

Ingredients:
1/3 cup of extra-virgin olive oil
1 tablespoon of mustard seeds
1 yellow onion, finely chopped
2 teaspoons of ginger, finely grated
2 medium garlic cloves, finely chopped
½ pound small potatoes, cubed
1-pound okra, thinly sliced
2 teaspoons of coriander
2 teaspoons of cumin
1 teaspoon of turmeric
1½ tablespoons of sesame seeds, toasted
½ teaspoon of red pepper, crushed
Salt to taste

Directions:

1. Heat up a pan with the olive oil, at a medium-high temperature. Cook mustard seeds for 15 seconds. Add onion. Cook for 2 more minutes. Stir occasionally.
2. Add garlic and ginger. Stir and cook for 2 minutes.
3. Add potatoes, salt, and red pepper. Stir. Cover. Cook for 5 minutes. Stir constantly.
4. Add okra, cumin, turmeric, and coriander. Stir and cook for 10 more minutes.
5. Add sesame seeds. Stir gently. Transfer onto plates. Serve!

Enjoy!

Nutritional value: 120 calories, 6 grams of fat, 10 grams of carbs, 2 grams of fiber, 2 grams of protein

Indian Style Okra

Try something new each night!

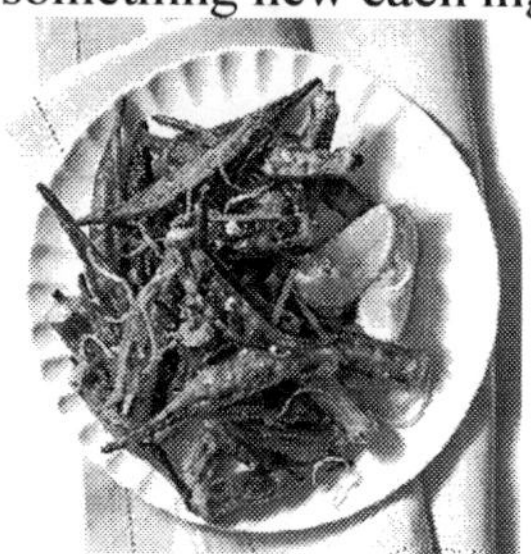

Ingredients:
2 tablespoons of extra-virgin olive oil
2 pounds of fresh okra
Zest of 2 limes
Juice from 2 limes
2 garlic cloves, finely chopped
1 lime cut into 8 wedges
1 tablespoon of garam masala
¼ cup of fresh cilantro, finely chopped
Salt and black pepper to taste

Directions:

1. In a bowl, mix okra with lime zest, lime juice, olive oil, garam masala, garlic, salt, and pepper. Stir well. Leave aside in a cool place or in the fridge for 1 hour.
2. Heat up your kitchen grill at a high temperature. Cook marinated okra for 10 minutes. Turn them occasionally.
3. Transfer okra onto plates. Season with salt and pepper if needed. Serve with chopped cilantro on top and lime wedges on the side.

Enjoy!

Nutritional value: 78 calories, 2 grams of fat, 8 grams of carbs, 3 grams of fiber, 2 grams of protein

Grilled Squash with Delicious Salsa

Simple and quick-to-make!

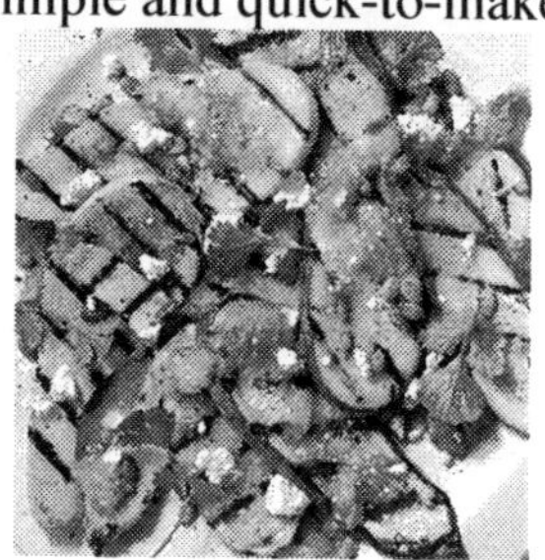

Ingredients:
3 tablespoons of extra-virgin olive oil
5 medium squash, sliced
1 cup of pepitas, unsalted and toasted
Sea salt to taste
¼ cup of goat cheese, crumbled
For the salsa:
7 tomatillos
Salt and black pepper to taste
1 small onion, finely chopped
2 tablespoons of fresh lime juice
2 tablespoons of fresh cilantro, chopped

Directions:

1. Heat up a pan at a medium temperature. Add tomatillos, onion and salt. Boil for 3 minutes. Take off heat. Drain. Transfer into your food processor. Leave them to cool down.
2. When tomatillos are cold, add lime juice and cilantro. Pulse a few times. Transfer into a small bowl. Leave aside for now.
3. Heat up your kitchen grill at a high temperature. Drizzle oil on squash slices. Grill them for 10 minutes.
4. Transfer squash onto serving plates. Add pepitas and goat cheese. Serve with the salsa you prepared earlier.

Enjoy!

Nutritional value: 80 calories, 2 grams of fat, 0 grams of carbs, 0 grams of fiber, 1 grams of protein

Dinner Salad with Tasty Garlic Dressing

This spicy salad is what you need for dinner tonight!

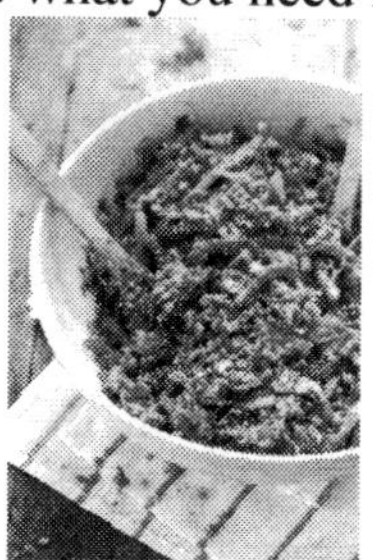

Ingredients:
1/3 cup of canola oil
1 tablespoon of sesame oil
2 tablespoons of cold water
3 tablespoons of soy sauce
2 tablespoons of vinegar
3 garlic cloves, minced
1 tablespoons of lemongrass paste
2 tablespoons of honey
½ teaspoon of lime juice
16 ounces of frozen edamame
6 cups of kale, chopped
1 red bell pepper, thinly sliced
1 yellow bell pepper, thinly sliced
3 carrots, thinly sliced
1 cup of cilantro leaves
3 green onions, thinly sliced
¾ cup of cashews
Salt and pepper to taste

Directions:

1. Mix canola oil with sesame oil, garlic, water, soy sauce, vinegar, lime juice, honey and lemongrass paste. Put this in your food processor. Pulse a few times. Transfer into a bowl. Leave aside.
2. Heat up a pot with water, at a medium-high temperature. Boil edamame for 5 minutes. Drain. Transfer into a bowl. Leave aside for 3 minutes.
3. In a large bowl, mix kale with carrots, bell peppers, cilantro, onions, and cashews.
4. Add edamame, salt, pepper and the salad dressing you prepared at the beginning. Serve!

Enjoy!

Nutritional value: 70 calories, 2 grams of fat, 7 grams of carbs, 1 gram of fiber, 2 grams of protein

Avocado Salad

This is an excellent dinner salad!

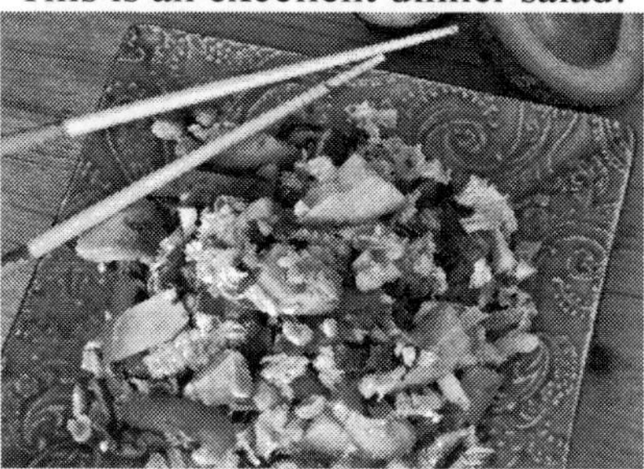

Ingredients:
1 small cabbage, finely chopped
1 cups of red cabbage, finely chopped
¼ cup of fresh mint, finely chopped
1 large avocado, cubed
1 orange bell pepper, thinly sliced
¼ cup of cilantro, chopped
1 tablespoon of fish sauce
¼ cup of peanuts, roasted and crushed
Juice from 2 limes
1 tablespoon of agave nectar

Directions:

1. In a bowl, mix cabbage with red cabbage, mint, bell pepper, avocado, and cilantro. Stir gently.
2. In another bowl, combine lime juice with agave nectar and fish sauce.
3. Add dressing to the salad. Toss to coat. Serve with peanuts on top.

Enjoy!

Nutritional value: 111 calories, 9 grams of fat, 8 grams of carbs, 4 grams of fiber, 1 grams of protein

Dinner Vegetarian Curry

Your next dinner!

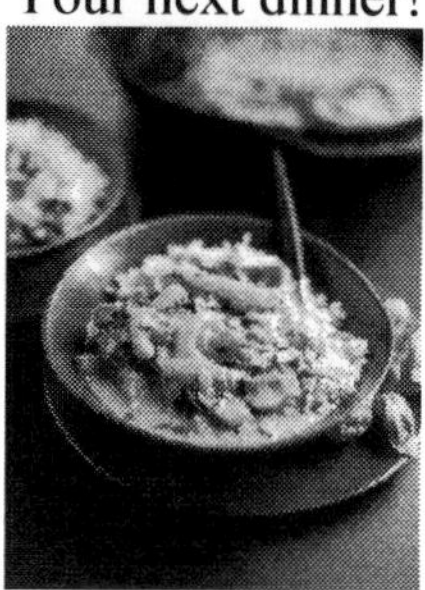

Ingredients:
1 tablespoon of coconut oil
1 yellow onion, finely chopped
1 cup of brown rice, rinsed
2 cups of water
1 tablespoon of grated ginger
2 garlic cloves, finely chopped
A pinch of salt
3 carrots, thinly sliced
1 red bell pepper, thinly sliced
1 yellow bell pepper, thinly sliced
1½ cups of kale, thinly sliced
2 tablespoons of curry paste
2 teaspoons of soy sauce
14 ounces of coconut milk
1½ teaspoons of rice vinegar
1½ teaspoons of coconut sugar
A sprigs basil, finely chopped

Directions:

1. Add 2 cups of water to a pot. Add the rice. Bring to a boil. Cook for 30 minutes. Stir occasionally. Drain. Transfer rice into a bowl. Leave aside for 10 minutes.
2. Heat up a saucepan with 1 tablespoon of oil, at a medium-high temperature. Add onion and some salt. Cook for 3-4 minutes. Stir constantly.
3. Add garlic and ginger. Cook for 1 minute.
4. Add carrots and peppers. Cook for 3-4 minutes more.
5. Add curry paste, coconut milk, kale, and coconut sugar. Bring to a boil. Cover. Reduce heat. Cook for 12 minutes.
6. Remove curry from heat. Add soy sauce and rice vinegar. Stir. Transfer onto serving plates. Serve with basil on top and with brown rice on the side.

Enjoy!

Nutritional value: 183 calories, 3 grams of fat, 16 grams of carbs, 6 grams of fiber, 5 grams of protein

Dinner Tofu Stew

The tofu will pick up the flavors of the other ingredients.

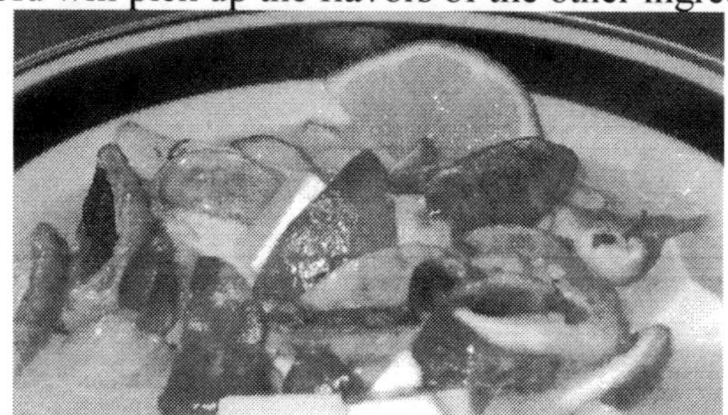

Ingredients:
14 ounces of coconut milk
12 ounces of firm tofu, cut into small pieces
2 cups of vegetable stock
5 lime leaves, shredded
2 tablespoons of lime juice
1-piece galangal
2 stalks lemongrass, chopped
½ teaspoon of red curry paste
½ cup of shiitake mushrooms, sliced
½ cup of button mushrooms, sliced
1/8 teaspoon of turmeric
2½ tablespoons of coconut sugar
4 ounces of rice noodles
½ teaspoon of red pepper flakes

Directions:

1. Put vegetable stock in a pot. Bring to a boil. Combine with coconut milk, galangal, lemongrass and lime leaves. Reduce to a simmer. Cook for 15 minutes.
2. Add tofu, curry paste, mushrooms, coconut sugar, lime juice and turmeric. Boil for another 10 minutes.
3. Cook the rice noodles according to the package instructions. Drain. Transfer them to serving plates. Add tofu stew on top. Sprinkle pepper flakes at the end.

Enjoy!

Nutritional value: 300 calories, 15 grams of fat, 20 grams of carbs, 0 grams of fiber, 10 grams of protein

Thai Vegan Pumpkin Stew

Here's a pumpkin stew you can have for dinner!

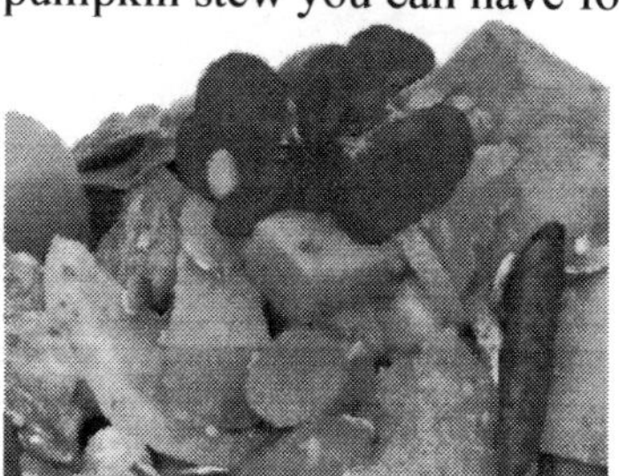

Ingredients:
1 squash, roughly chopped
1 potato, roughly chopped
2 carrots, thinly sliced
1 cup of cherry tomatoes, halved
1 yellow bell pepper, sliced
2 red chilies, finely chopped
½ can chickpeas, drained
10 ounces of coconut milk
2 tablespoons of orange rind, grated
4 garlic cloves, crushed
1 teaspoon of tamarind paste
2 and ½ tablespoons of soy sauce
1 tablespoon of coconut sugar
1/3 purple onion, finely chopped
½ teaspoon of turmeric
1 tablespoon of coriander seeds
1 tablespoon of cider vinegar
1 teaspoon of fennel seeds, 1 tablespoon of cumin, and 1 teaspoon of pumpkin seeds
½ small bunch fresh basil, finely chopped

Directions:

1. In a bowl, mix garlic with chilies, tamarind paste, coconut milk, soy sauce, sugar, lime juice, orange juice, turmeric, vinegar, purple onion, coriander, and cumin and fennel seeds. Put this mix into your food processor. Pulse a few times. Transfer to a bowl again. Leave aside for now.
2. Heat up a pan at a medium-high temperature. Add squash, potato, carrots and the curry paste you made earlier. Stir and cook for 8 minutes. Add chickpeas, tomatoes and bell pepper. Cook for another 2 minutes.
3. Transfer onto serving plates. Sprinkle chopped basil and pumpkin seeds on top.

Enjoy!

Nutritional value: 250 calories, 8 grams of fat, 20 grams of carbs, 3 grams of fiber, 16 grams of protein

Broccoli and Quinoa Dish

It's one of the best dishes you'll have!

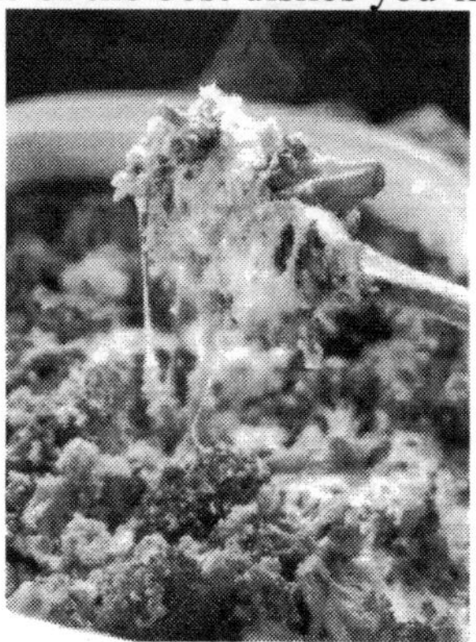

Ingredients:
2 and ½ cups of quinoa
4 and ½ cups of vegetable stock
½ teaspoon of salt
2 tablespoons of pesto sauce
2 tablespoons of arrowroot powder
12 ounces of mozzarella cheese
2 cups of spinach
12 ounces of broccoli
1/3 cup of parmesan
3 green onions, finely chopped

Directions:

1. Put quinoa and green onions into a baking dish. Leave aside.
2. Put broccoli in a heatproof bowl. Put food in the microwave. Cook on high for 5 minutes. Then leave to the side.
3. In a bowl, mix vegetable stock with arrowroot powder, pesto sauce, and some salt. Stir well. Transfer into a pot. Bring to a boil.
4. Pour this over quinoa. Add broccoli, spinach, parmesan and almost all the mozzarella cheese.
5. Put food into the oven at 400 degrees F. Bake for 30 minutes.
6. Take the dish of the oven. Sprinkle the rest of the cheese. Bake for 5 more minutes.
7. Take out of the oven again. Leave aside for 2-3 minutes. Transfer onto plates. Serve.

Enjoy!

Nutritional value: 420 calories, 16 grams of fat, 61 grams of carbs, 9 grams of fiber, 27 grams of protein

Delicate Dinner Salad

It's going to transform your dinner into a feast!

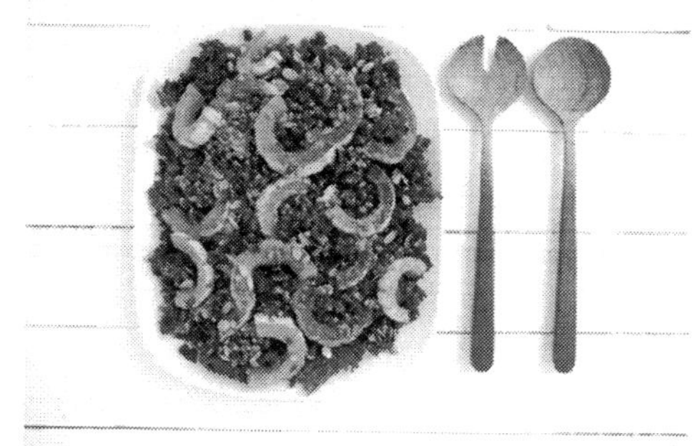

Ingredients:
1 medium squash, halved lengthwise and sliced
3 tablespoons of extra-virgin olive oil
Salt and black pepper to taste
1/4 cup of orange juice
Zest from 1 orange
1 tablespoon of white wine vinegar
1 tablespoon of maple syrup
2 bunches kale leaves, torn into small pieces
1/2 cup of pomegranate seeds
1/4 cup of wheat berries, cooked according to instructions
1/4 cup of pepitas

Directions:

1. In a bowl, mix squash with 1 tablespoon of oil. Transfer it onto a baking sheet. Season with salt and pepper. Put food in the oven at 400 degrees F. Bake for about 20 minutes.
2. Meanwhile, in a bowl, mix the rest of the olive oil with orange juice, vinegar, maple syrup, orange zest, and salt and pepper to taste. Stir well.
3. Put kale leaves in a bowl. Add baked squash, pomegranate seeds, wheat berries, and pepitas. Drizzle the vinaigrette on top.

Enjoy!

Nutritional value: 170 calories, 20 grams of fat, 15 grams of carbs, 6 grams of fiber, 4 grams of protein

Vegetarian Pad Thai

It's going to become one of your favorites!

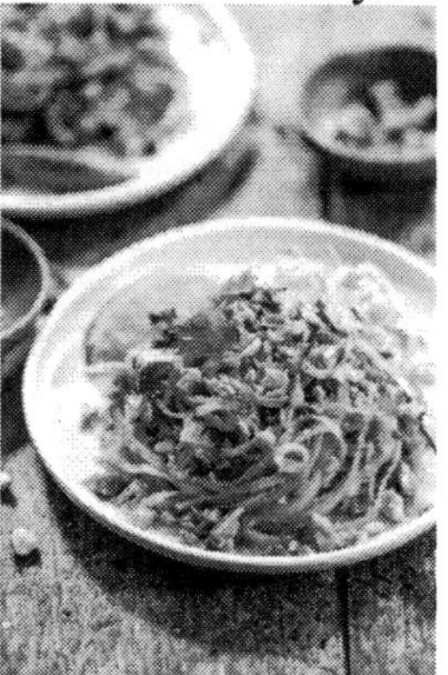

Ingredients:
For the Pad Thai:
4 ounces of brown rice noodles
1 zucchini, thinly sliced
1 red pepper, thinly sliced
½ yellow onion, thinly sliced
2 carrots, thinly sliced
2 tablespoons of extra-virgin olive oil
1 egg whisked
½ cup of peanuts, roughly chopped
½ cup of fresh cilantro, green onions, and basil, mixed and finely chopped
For the Sauce:
3 tablespoons of vegan fish sauce
3 tablespoons of coconut sugar
3 tablespoons of vegetable broth
2 tablespoons of white vinegar
1 tablespoon of soy sauce
1 teaspoon of chili paste

Directions:

1. Place noodles in a bowl. Add water. Soak for a few minutes. Drain. Leave aside.
2. Heat up a pan with 1 tablespoon of oil, at a medium-high temperature. Add vegetables. Cook for 3 minutes. Stir constantly. Transfer to a dish. Leave aside.
3. Heat up 1 more tablespoon of oil in the pan. Add noodles. Cook for 1 minute. Add sauce. Stir. Cook for another minute or two.
4. Pour the egg into the pan. Cook for 30 seconds. Stir gently. Toss everything around with the tongs. Add the vegetables. Toss to coat. Remove from heat. Add peanuts and mixed herbs. Transfer onto plates. Serve.

Enjoy!

Nutritional value: 376 calories, 18 grams of fat, 44 grams of carbs, 5 grams of fiber, 12 grams of protein

Vegetarian Dinner Gazpacho

It's an elegant and creamy choice for dinner!

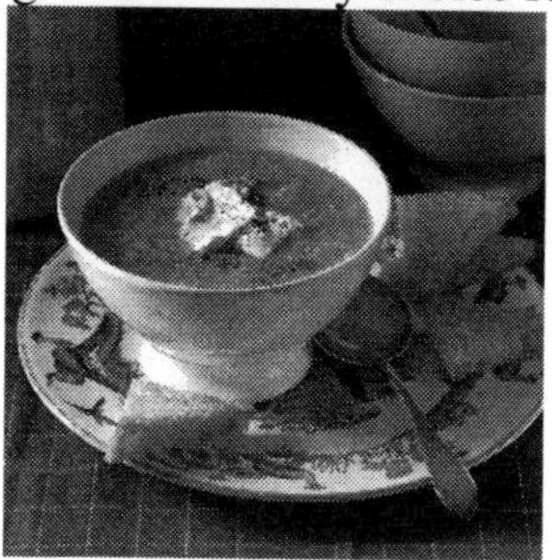

Ingredients:
1 pound of yellow tomatoes, chopped
1 yellow bell pepper, chopped
1 yellow squash, chopped
2 shallots, finely chopped
1 cup of fresh carrot juice
2 tablespoons of sherry wine vinegar
¾ teaspoon of salt
½ cup of fresh mint leaves, finely chopped

Directions:

1. In your food processor, mix tomatoes with squash, bell pepper, shallots, salt, vinegar and carrot juice. Pulse a few times.
2. Transfer into a bowl. Keep in the fridge for now.
3. Meanwhile, heat up a pan with some water, at a medium temperature. Add mint. Leave for 10 seconds. Drain. Leave aside.
4. Take soup out of the fridge. Pour into serving bowls. Serve with mint on top,

Enjoy!

Nutritional value: 60 calories, 1 gram of fat, 14 grams of carbs, 2 grams of fiber, 2 grams of protein

Dinner Pea Salad

It's super delicious!

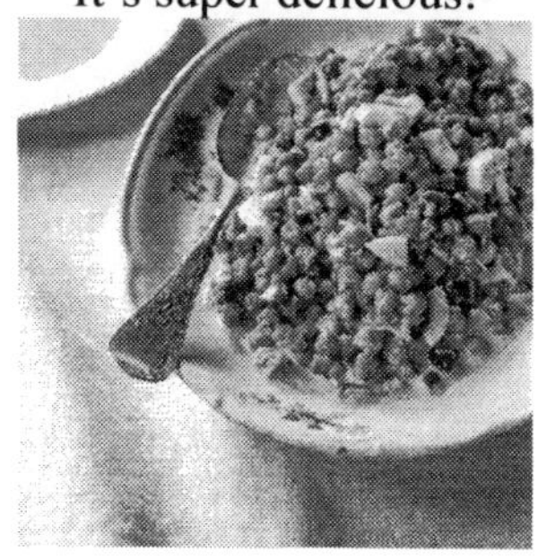

Ingredients:
2 eggs, already boiled and sliced
60 ounces of peas
1 yellow bell pepper, chopped
2 ounces of Cheddar cheese, grated
½ cup of vegetarian mayonnaise
3 tablespoons of dried basil
2 tablespoons of red onion, finely chopped
2 teaspoons of pimiento, finely chopped
1 teaspoon of apple cider vinegar
1 teaspoon of coconut sugar
Salt and black pepper to taste
1 teaspoon of garlic powder
A drizzle of hot sauce

Directions:

1. In a salad bowl, mix egg slices with bell pepper, cheese, onion, basil, pimiento, salt, and pepper. Stir.
2. Add mayo, sugar, vinegar, hot sauce and garlic powder. Stir.
3. Add peas. Toss well. Put in the fridge. Serve cold!

Enjoy!

Nutritional value: 230 calories, 20 grams of fat, 15 grams of carbs, 8 grams of fiber, 12 grams of protein

Special Dinner Pasta

It's a very tasty dish with wonderful flavors!

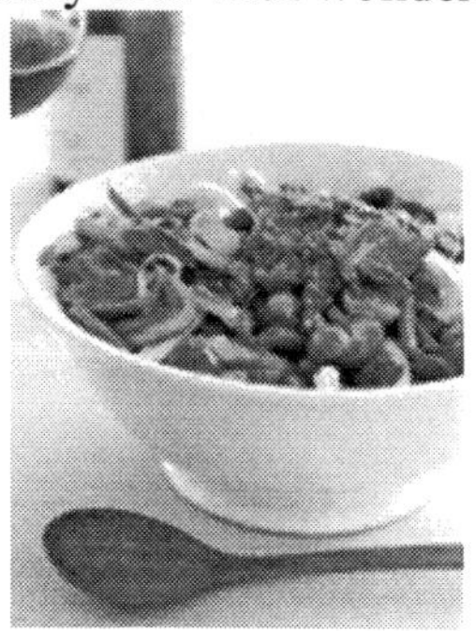

Ingredients:
½ cup of extra-virgin olive oil
1 tablespoon of extra-virgin olive oil
½ pound cranberry beans
3 cups of basil leaves, finely chopped
5 tablespoons of fresh lemon juice
2 garlic cloves, finely chopped
¾ cup of Parmesan cheese, finely grated
¾ pound pasta
8 ounces of green beans
1 yellow onion, finely chopped
⅓ cup of white wine
8 ounces of grape tomatoes

Directions:

1. Put beans in a pot. Cover with water. Bring to a boil over a medium-high temperature. Then remove from heat. Cover. Leave aside for 1 hour.
2. Drain beans. Discard water. Return them to pot. Add some water. Season with some salt. Bring to a boil again. Reduce heat to medium. Boil for 45 minutes.
3. Drain again. Reserve liquid. Transfer beans into a bowl. Leave aside. Keep warm.
4. In a bowl, mix basil with 1 garlic clove, lemon juice, parmesan, and salt and pepper to taste. Stir. Put mix into your food processor. Pulse a few times. Add ½ cup of oil. Pulse. Leave aside.
5. Cook pasta according to package instructions. Drain. Leave aside.
6. Heat up the rest of the oil in a pan at a medium-high temperature. Cook the rest of the garlic for 30 seconds. Add onion. Cook for 7 minutes. Add beans, salt, pepper, wine, green beans and some of the liquid left over from boiling the beans. Stir and cook for 3 more minutes.
7. Put pasta on serving plates. Add bean mix and the basil pesto you prepared earlier. Serve with tomatoes on top.

Enjoy!

Nutritional value: 250 calories, 3 grams of fat, 17 grams of carbs, 1 gram of fiber, 9 grams of proteins

Fennel and Apple Salad

It can be both a tasty dinner and a successful side salad! It's your choice!

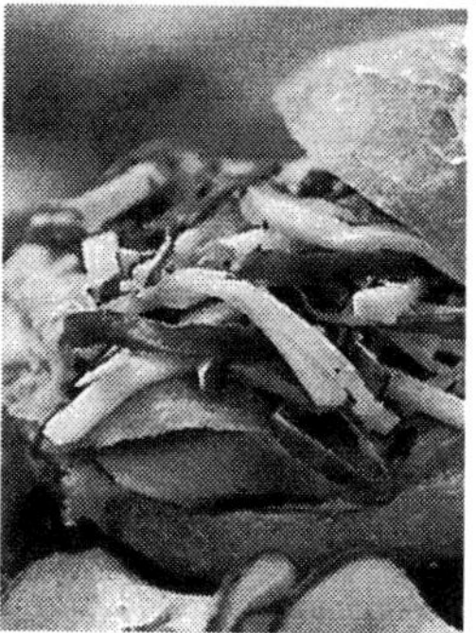

Ingredients:
4 cups of red cabbage, shredded
2 large apples, sliced
1½ cup of fennel, shredded
1/3 cup of coconut yogurt
1/3 cup of vegan mayonnaise
3 tablespoons of apple cider vinegar
½ teaspoon of caraway seeds
½ teaspoon of palm sugar
Black pepper to taste

Directions:

1. In a bowl, mix fennel with cabbage and apples.
2. In another bowl, mix coconut yogurt with mayo, vinegar, sugar, black pepper and caraway seeds. Stir well.
3. Pour this over salad. Toss to coat. Keep in the fridge until you serve it!

Enjoy!

Nutritional value: 160 calories, 4 grams of fat, 10 grams of carbs, 6 grams of fiber, 3 grams of protein

Tasty Roasted Celery

It's going to be one of the best dinners you've ever had!

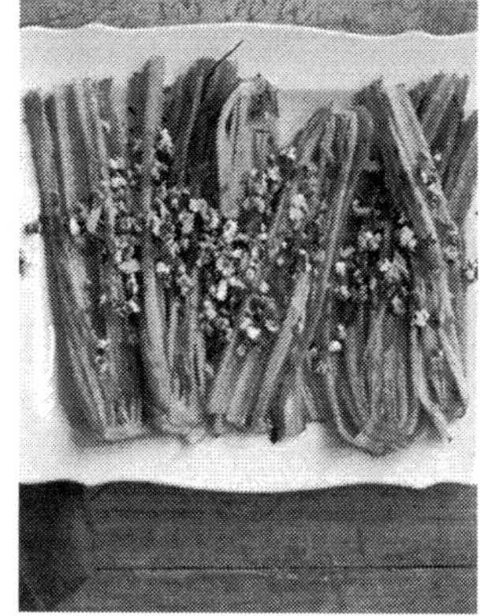

Ingredients:
3 bunches celery, halved
1 celery, cubed
2 tablespoons of extra-virgin olive oil
Salt and black pepper to taste
2 cups of apple juice
5 tablespoons of honey
5 ounces of blue cheese
¼ cup of parsley, finely chopped
¼ cup of walnuts

Directions:

1. Put water in a pot. Bring to a boil. Add salt and celery halves. Boil for 3 minutes. Drain. Transfer into a baking pan.
2. Add oil, 3 tablespoons of honey, salt, apple juice and pepper. Put food in the oven at 450 degrees F. Bake for 25 minutes.
3. Take celery out of the oven. Transfer to a platter. Leave aside.
4. In a bowl, mix blue cheese with pepper, some salt, walnuts, parsley and the rest of the celery.
5. Add this to baked celery. Drizzle the rest of the honey on top. Serve!

Enjoy!

Nutritional value: 130 calories, 5 grams of fat, 3 grams of carbs, 1 gram of fiber, 6 grams of protein

Roasted Spring Onions

It's probably the easiest dinner recipe ever!

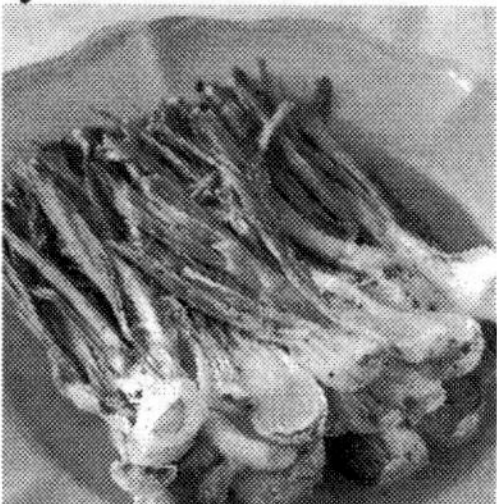

Ingredients:
15 spring onions
Salt and black pepper to taste
1 teaspoon of thyme, chopped
1 tablespoon of unsalted coconut butter

Directions:

1. Put onions in a baking dish. Add thyme on top. Season with salt and pepper.
2. Add butter. Put food in the oven at 350 degrees F. Bake for 40 minutes.
3. Take out of the oven. Transfer to a serving platter. Drizzle juices from the pan over onions. Serve!

Enjoy!

Nutritional value: 70 calories, 2 grams of fat, 7 grams of carbs, 3 grams of fiber, 2 grams of protein

Delicious Mashed Potatoes

The taste is really subtle! You'll love this dish!

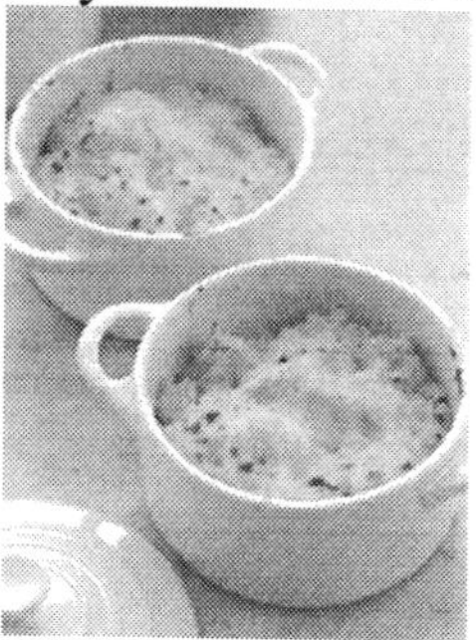

Ingredients:
2 pounds of gold potatoes, cut into small pieces
1½ cup of fresh ricotta cheese
Sea salt and black pepper to taste
½ cup of almond milk
3 tablespoons of coconut butter

Directions:

1. Put potatoes in a pot. Cover with salted water. Place on stove over medium temperature. Bring to a boil. Cook for 20 minutes.
2. Drain potatoes, return all the potatoes to the pot and mash them except for 1 cup of the potatoes. Add salt, pepper, milk, butter and ricotta to the mashed potatoes. Stir well.
3. Add the rest of the 1 cup of potatoes. Mash again.
4. Spoon mashed potatoes in 10 ramekins. Place them into a baking pan. Broil them until they change their color.
5. Serve hot!

Enjoy!

Nutritional value: 180 calories, 9 grams of fat, 18 grams of carbs, 1 gram of fiber, 7 grams of protein

Amazing Potato Salad

This salad is truly amazing!

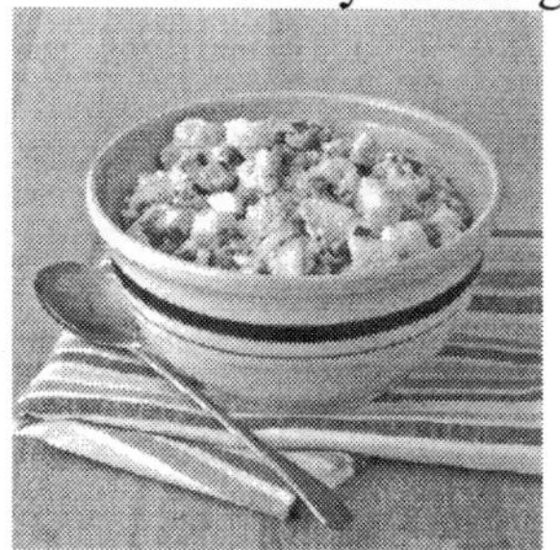

Ingredients:
3 pounds of red potatoes
¾ cup of red pepper, chopped
¾ cup of white onion, chopped
¾ cup of celery, chopped
3 eggs hard boiled and, chopped
½ cup of dill pickles, finely chopped
2 tablespoons of dill pickle juice
¾ cup of vegan mayo
1 tablespoon of cider vinegar
Salt and black pepper

Directions:

1. Put potatoes in a pot. Cover with salted water. Place on the stove. Bring to a boil over a high temperature. Cook for 40 minutes. Drain. Cut in pieces. Transfer into a bowl. Keep warm.
2. In a bowl, mix white onion with celery, red pepper, dill pickles, eggs, potatoes, vinegar and pickle juice. Stir.
3. Add vegan mayo, and salt and pepper to taste. Toss to coat. Cool in the fridge before you serve it.

Enjoy!

Nutritional value: 340 calories, 20 grams of fat, 27 grams of carbs, 6 grams of protein

Grilled Vegetables with Special Glaze

A light dinner for you to enjoy with your loved ones!

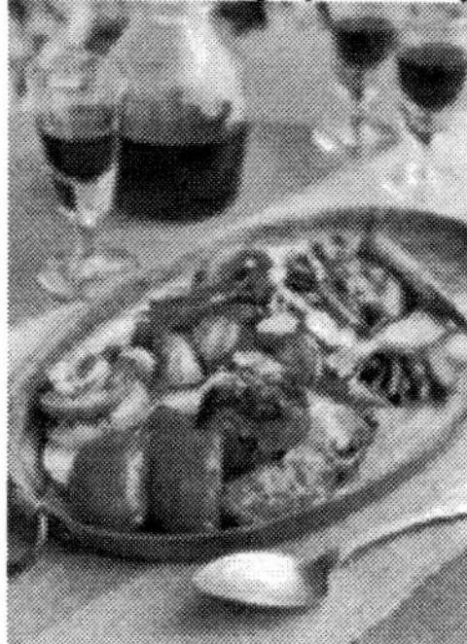

Ingredients:
2 pounds of mixed tomatoes, carrots and radishes
1/3 cup of red wine
1/3 cup of balsamic vinegar
Salt and black pepper to taste
2 tablespoons of extra-virgin olive oil
1 spring summer savory

Directions:

1. In a bowl, mix red wine with balsamic vinegar. Pour into a pot. Bring to a boil over a medium-high temperature. Reduce heat. Simmer for 25 minutes until you obtain a ¼ cup of balsamic glaze.
2. Mix vegetables with olive oil. Season them with salt and pepper to taste. Place on heated grill. Cook carrots and radishes for 10 minutes, and tomatoes for 2 minutes on each side.
3. Transfer vegetables onto a platter. Drizzle glaze on top. Sprinkle summer savory at the end.

Enjoy!

Nutritional value: 120 calories, 1 gram of fat, 9 grams of carbs, 2 grams of fiber, 2 grams of protein

Vegetable Croquettes

Oh my God! These taste so great!

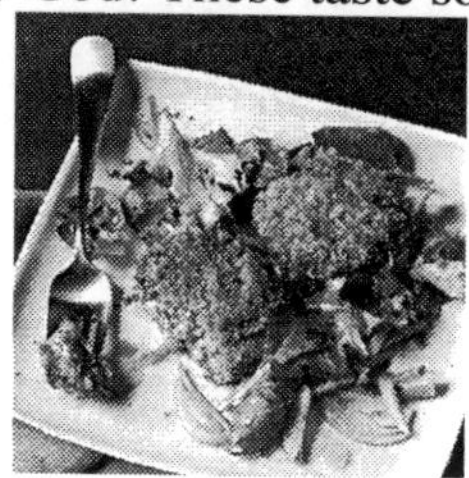

Ingredients:
8 ounces of potatoes
4 ounces of button mushrooms, sliced
4 ounces of cremini mushrooms, sliced
Cooking spray
½ leek, chopped
1 teaspoon of thyme, chopped
1 ounce of parmesan cheese
2 ounces of gruyere cheese, shredded
Salt and black pepper to taste
1 egg yolk
1 egg white
2 teaspoons of water
½ cup of breadcrumbs
1 tablespoon of extra-virgin olive oil
1/3 cup of almond flour

Directions:

1. Put potatoes in a pot. Cover with water. Bring to a boil over a high heat. Reduce temperature. Simmer for 8 minutes. Drain. Mash them roughly. Place them into a bowl. Leave aside.
2. In your food processor, mix leek with thyme and mushrooms. Pulse them a few times.
3. Heat up a pan after spraying it with some oil, at a medium heat. Add mushroom mix. Cook for 6 minutes. Stir occasionally.
4. Mix this with potatoes. Add gruyere, half of the parmesan, salt, pepper and egg yolk. Stir well.
5. Shape 8 patties from this mix. Place them on a plate.
6. In another dish, mix 2 teaspoons of water with egg white. Whisk well.
7. In a third dish, mix breadcrumbs with the rest of the parmesan.
8. Dredge each of the patties in flour, then dip them in the egg and breadcrumb mix. Heat up a pan with the olive oil, at a high temperature. Add patties. Cook for 4 minutes on each side.
9. Transfer them to a platter. Serve right away!

Enjoy!

Nutritional value: 266 calories, 10 grams of fat, 29 grams of carbs, 2 grams of fiber, 12 grams of protein

Delicious Farfalle with Tomatoes

Make everyone happy at dinnertime with this delicious recipe!

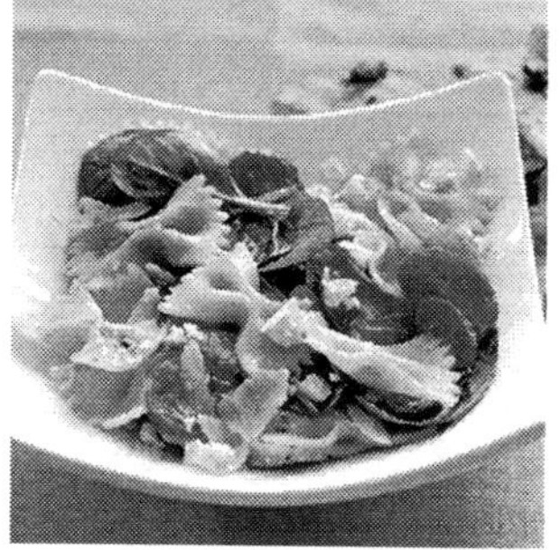

Ingredients:
8 ounces of farfalle pasta
2 tablespoons of extra-virgin olive oil
1 yellow onion, sliced
1 teaspoon of dried oregano
Salt and black pepper to taste
2 cups of grape tomatoes, cut in halves
5 garlic cloves, sliced
1 tablespoon of white wine vinegar
3 tablespoons of parmesan cheese
3 cups of baby spinach
3 ounces of feta cheese, crumbled

Directions:

1. Put water in a pot. Add some salt. Bring to a boil. Add pasta. Cook according to package instructions. Drain. Leave aside.
2. Heat up a pan with 1 tablespoon of oil, at a medium-high temperature. Add onion. Cook for 10 minutes.
3. Add oregano. Stir and cook for 2 more minutes.
4. Add garlic. Cook for another 2 minutes.
5. Add vinegar and tomatoes. Stir and cook for 3 minutes.
6. Add spinach and pasta. Stir and cook for 1 minute.
7. Remove from heat. Add parmesan, salt and pepper to taste, and the rest of the oil. Toss to coat.
8. Transfer onto plates. Serve with feta cheese sprinkled on top.

Enjoy!

Nutritional value: 374 calories, 13 grams of fat, 51 grams of carbs, 3 grams of fiber,

Vegetarian Stuffed Potatoes

You'll forget about simple baked potatoes in no time once you try this recipe!

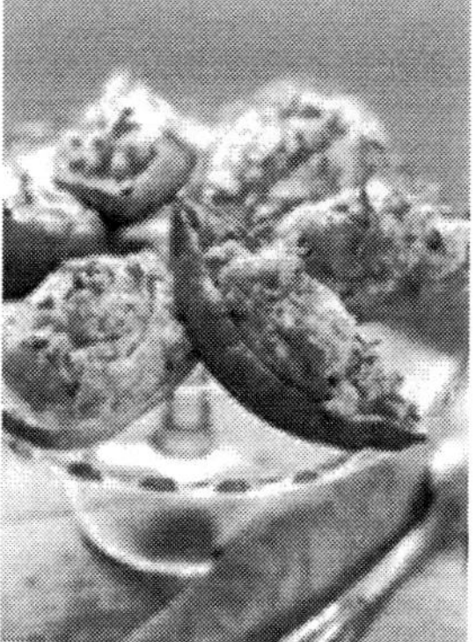

Ingredients:
2 pears, roughly chopped
Juice from 1 lemon
4 medium potatoes, baked
5 tablespoons of unsalted butter
1 egg
½ cup of almond milk
13 cloves ground
Salt and black pepper
¼ teaspoon of nutmeg, grated
½ cup of palm sugar
3 sprigs thyme, finely chopped

Directions:

1. Put pears in a pot. Cover with water. Bring to a boil. Add lemon juice. Reduce heat. Cook for 15 minutes, then remove food from the pan. Leave aside for now.
2. Cut baked potatoes in half. Scoop flesh. Place in a bowl. Reserve potato skins.
3. Mix potatoes flesh with milk, butter, and pears. Mash everything.
4. Add cloves, salt, pepper, egg, and half of the nutmeg. Stir again.
5. Fill egg skins with this mix. Place them on a lined baking sheet. Sprinkle the rest of the nutmeg, and the sugar and thyme on top. Put food in the oven at 425 degrees F. Bake for 25 minutes.
6. Take potatoes out of the oven. Leave them to cool down. Transfer onto plates. Serve!

Enjoy!

Nutritional value: 120 calories, 30 grams of fat, 28 grams of carbs, 20 grams of fiber, 18 grams of protein

Dinner Mix

It's a dinner mix to suit all tastes!

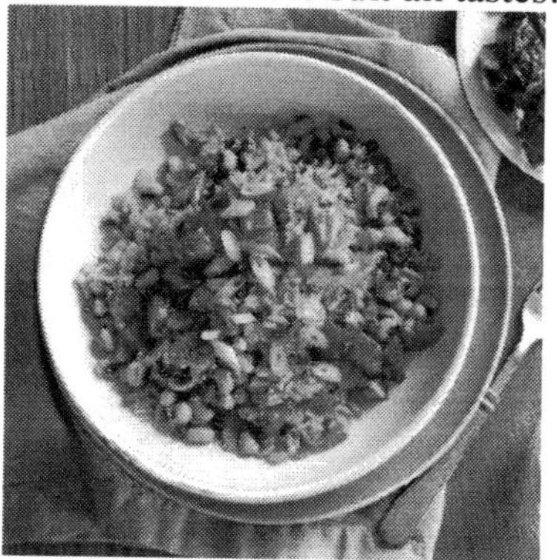

Ingredients:
1½ cups of yellow onion, finely chopped
1½ cups of red bell pepper, finely chopped
5 teaspoons of extra-virgin olive oil
1 cup of celery, thinly sliced
1 tablespoon of garlic, minced
¾ cup of vegetable stock
½ cup of brown rice
½ cup of water
Salt and black pepper to taste
½ teaspoon of thyme, chopped
¾ teaspoon of paprika
¼ teaspoon of ground red pepper
1/3 cup of tomato, chopped
4 teaspoons of green onions, finely chopped
45 ounces of canned black peas, drained

Directions:

1. Heat up a pan with the oil, at a medium-high temperature. Add onion, celery and bell pepper. Stir and cook for 7 minutes.
2. Add garlic. Cook 1 more minute.
3. Add rice, stock, water, salt, pepper, paprika, thyme and red pepper. Stir. Bring to a boil. Reduce heat. Cover. Simmer for 10 minutes.
4. Add peas. Stir and cook for 2 more minutes.
5. Add tomato and green onions. Stir gently. Transfer onto plates. Serve!

Enjoy!

Nutritional value: 287 calories, 7 grams of fat, 45 grams of carbs, 10 grams of fiber, 12 grams of protein

Potato Pancakes

Easy to make!

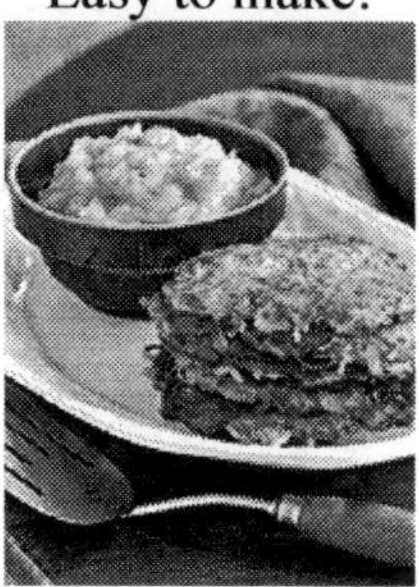

Ingredients:
1 yellow onion, finely chopped
1 pound of russet potatoes, grated
Salt and black pepper to taste
2 and ½ teaspoons of grated nutmeg
2 tablespoons of almond flour
1 egg
1½ tablespoons of canola oil

Directions:

1. In a bowl, mix potatoes with salt, onion, nutmeg, pepper, flour and egg. Stir well.
2. Heat up ¾ tablespoon of oil in a pan at a medium-high temperature. Put 3 tablespoons of potato mix in the pan. Flatten the mix with a spatula. Reduce heat. Cook each side of the potatoes for 5 minutes.
3. Repeat this with the rest of the batter and the oil. Transfer all pancakes on a platter. Serve warm!

Enjoy!

Nutritional value: 70 calories, 2 grams of fat, 10 grams of carbs, 1 grams of fiber, 1 grams of protein

Barley Salad

It's a creamy salad you should try soon!

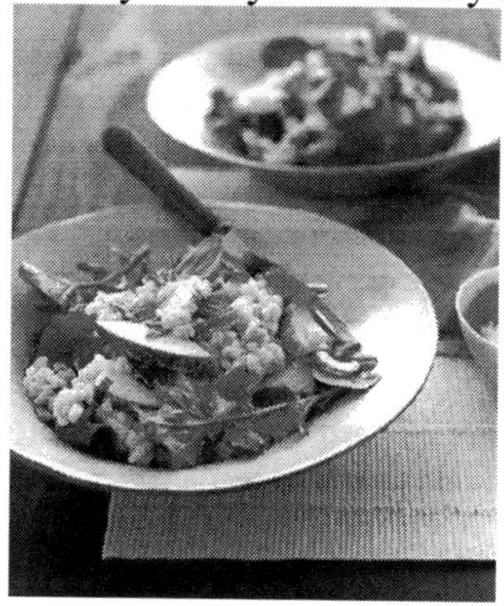

Ingredients:
½ cup of barley
1½ cup of water
½ cup of coconut yogurt
Salt and black pepper to taste
2 tablespoons of extra-virgin olive oil
1 teaspoon of mustard
1 tablespoon of lemon juice
2 celery stalks, sliced
¼ cup of mint, finely chopped
1 apple thinly, sliced
2 bunches arugula, stems removed

Directions:

1. Put barley in a pan. Add the water and some salt. Bring to a boil. Reduce heat. Cover. Simmer for 25 minutes. Drain. Spread on a baking sheet. Leave aside.
2. In a bowl, mix yogurt with lemon juice, oil, salt, pepper, and mustard. Stir well.
3. Add mint, apple, celery, and barley. Toss to coat.
4. Divide arugula in 4 bowls. Add barley mix on top. Serve!

Enjoy!

Nutritional value: 198 calories, 8 grams of fat, 29 grams of carbs, 6 grams of fiber, 5 grams of protein

Greens with Artichoke Vinaigrette

Simple yet surprising in taste!

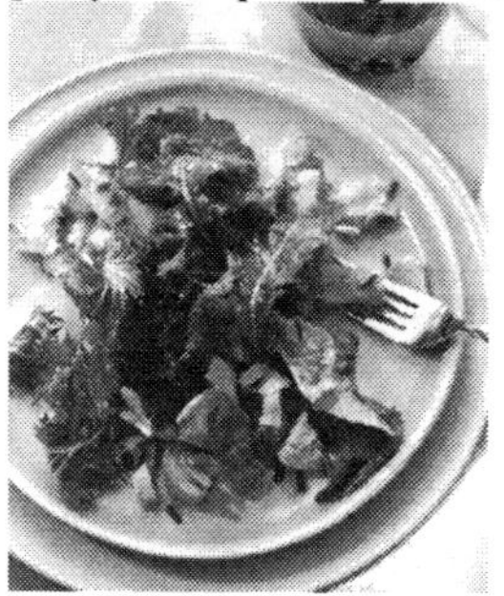

Ingredients:
12 ounces of jarred artichokes hearts, drained and chopped
3 tablespoons of lemon juice
1/3 cup of extra-virgin olive oil
10 ounces of mixed greens
Salt and black pepper to taste

Directions:

1. In a bowl, mix lemon juice with artichokes, salt, pepper, and oil. Stir well.
2. Divide greens on serving plates. Add artichoke vinaigrette. Toss to coat. Serve right away!

Enjoy!

Nutritional value: 112 calories, 9 grams of fat, 6 grams of carbs, 2 grams of fiber, 2 grams of protein

Delightful Dinner

It's something you never had before! We are sure!

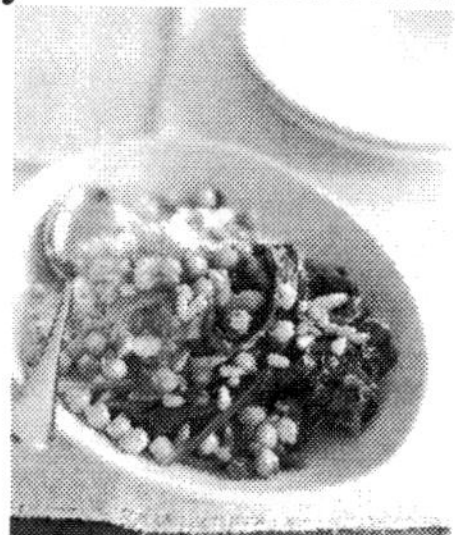

Ingredients:
10 ounces of couscous
1½ cup of boiling water
½ cup of pine nuts
2 garlic cloves, finely chopped
3 tablespoons of extra-virgin olive oil
15 ounces of canned chickpeas rinsed
½ cup of raisins
2 bunches Swiss chard, trimmed
Salt and black pepper to taste

Directions:

1. Put the couscous in a bowl. Add water. Stir. Cover. Leave aside for 10 minutes.
2. Meanwhile, heat up a pan at a medium-high temperature. Add pine nuts. Toast them for 4 minutes. Transfer onto a plate. Leave aside.
3. Return the pan to heat. Add oil. Heat up. Add garlic. Stir and cook for 1 minute.
4. Add raisins, chickpeas, chard, salt and pepper. Stir and cook for 5 minutes.
5. Fluff couscous. Divide on serving plates. Add chard and chickpeas mix. Top with pine nuts. Serve!

Enjoy!

Nutritional value: 540 calories, 24 grams of fat, 71 grams of carbs, 13 grams of fiber, 17 grams of protein

Vegetable Sheppard's Pie

Are you willing to try a whole different version of the classic Sheppard's Pie?

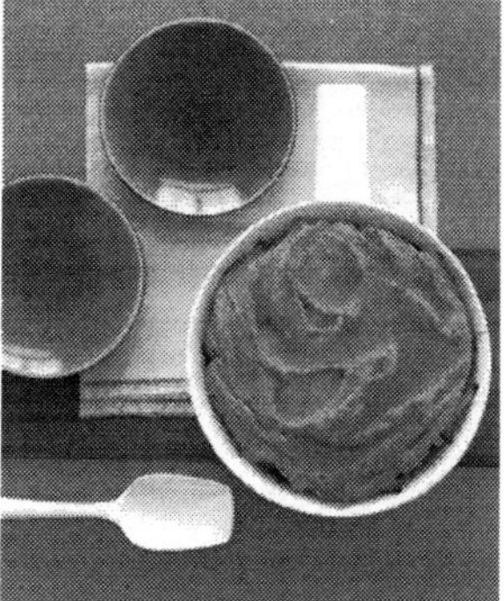

Ingredients:
2 pounds of potatoes, cut in chunks
6 tablespoons of unsalted butter
Salt and black pepper to taste
2 parsnips, sliced
1 yellow onion, thinly sliced
2 medium fennel bulbs, diced
2 celery stalks, sliced
2 tablespoons of parsley, finely chopped
2 cups of Brussels sprouts, cut in halves
15 ounces of vegetable stock
3 cups of fresh spinach
A pinch of nutmeg

Directions:

1. Put potatoes in a pot. Add some salt. Cover with water. Bring to a boil. Reduce heat. Simmer for 20 minutes. Drain. Leave aside for now.
2. Heat up a pan with 2 tablespoons of butter, at a medium-high temperature. Add onion. Cook for 10 minutes. Stir occasionally.
3. Add celery, fennel, parsnips, parsley, Brussels sprouts, salt and pepper. Stir.
4. Add stock. Simmer for 15 minutes. Add spinach. Stir. Remove from heat.
5. Transfer vegetable mix into a casserole. Leave aside for now.
6. Transfer potatoes into a pot. Heat them up. Add the rest of the butter. Mash potatoes and add them on top of the vegetables. Place food in your broiler. Cook for 5 minutes. Sprinkle nutmeg on top. Serve!

Enjoy!

Nutritional value: 235 calories, 9 grams of fat, 37 grams of carbs, 8 grams of fiber, 5 grams of protein

Spinach and Ricotta Gnocchi

Cook this Italian dish for your next dinner!

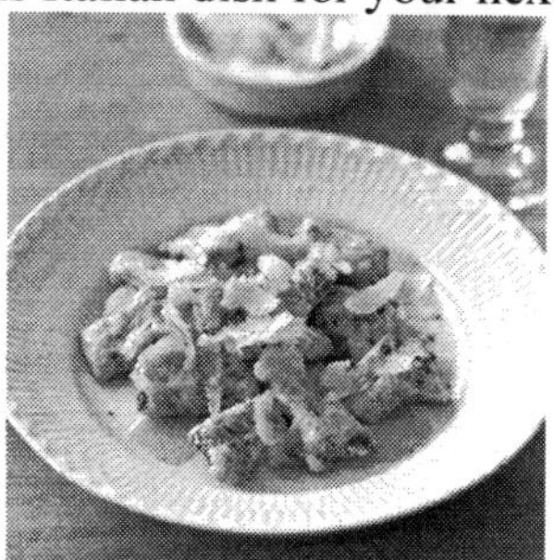

Ingredients:
1 package of frozen spinach
2 egg yolks
2 eggs
Salt and black pepper to taste
16 ounces of ricotta cheese
1 cup of parmesan grated
¼ teaspoon of nutmeg
1 cup of almond flour
A drizzle of extra-virgin olive oil

Directions:

1. In a bowl, mix eggs with spinach, egg yolks, salt, pepper, ricotta, parmesan, nutmeg, and flour. Stir well.
2. Shape ropes from the batter. Cut them into pieces and place them on a working surface.
3. Put some water in a pot. Add some salt. Bring to a boil. Add spinach gnocchi you prepared earlier. Cook for 4 minutes.
4. Drain them. Transfer onto plates. Drizzle some olive oil on top. Serve!

Enjoy!

Nutritional value: 230 calories, 10 grams of fat, 23 grams of carbs, 3 grams of fiber, 21 grams of protein

Wonderful Bread Salad

Something you never ate before!

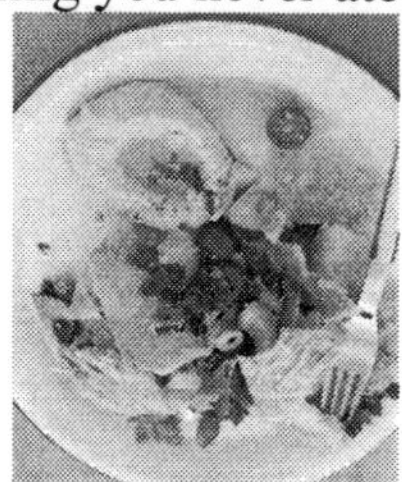

Ingredients:
1 cucumber, thinly sliced
2 stale pitas, split
14 cherry tomatoes, cut in halves
1 fennel bulb, chopped
3 scallions thinly, sliced
2 celery stalks, chopped
2 tablespoons of mint, finely chopped
¼ cup of extra-virgin olive oil
½ cup of parsley, finely chopped
Juice from 1 lemon
Salt and black pepper to taste
1 garlic clove, finely chopped

Directions:

1. Put pita rounds on a baking sheet. Put food in the oven at 350 degrees F. Bake for 10 minutes. Take out of the oven. Break them in pieces. Leave aside for now.
2. Meanwhile, in a bowl, mix tomatoes with cucumber, fennel, scallions, mint, celery and parsley. Cover. Keep in the fridge for now.
3. In another bowl, mix lemon juice with, oil, garlic, and salt and pepper to taste. Stir well.
4. Take vegetables out of the fridge. Add salad dressing. Toss to coat. Arrange on plates. Serve with pita pieces on top.

Enjoy!

Nutritional value: 264 calories, 14 grams of fat, 31 grams of carbs, 5 grams of fiber, 6 grams of protein

Tomato Burger

A tasty summer "burger"

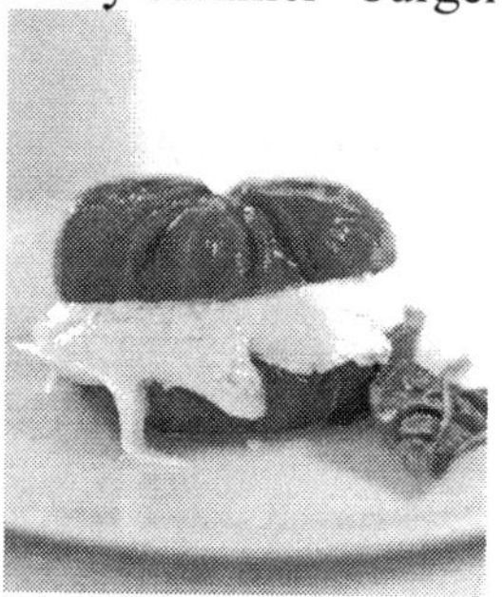

Ingredients:
6 large tomatoes
Salt and black pepper to taste
2 tablespoons of olive oil
1 garlic clove, thinly sliced
2 basil sprigs, roughly chopped
8 ounces of unsalted mozzarella, sliced

Directions:

1. Slice a piece from the bottom of tomatoes. Slice them in half horizontally. Place them on a baking sheet.
2. Season them with salt and pepper. Drizzle the oil on top.
3. Add garlic slices over tomatoes. Put food in the oven at 450 degrees F. Bake for 15 minutes.
4. Take tomatoes out of the oven. Place a mozzarella slice between 2 tomato halves. Transfer onto a plate. Drizzle pan juices over them. Serve with basil on top.

Enjoy!

Nutritional value: 182 calories, 6 grams of fat, 8 grams of carbs, 2 grams of fiber, 8 grams of protein

Vegetable Noodles and Tasty Coconut Sauce

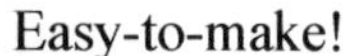
Easy-to-make!

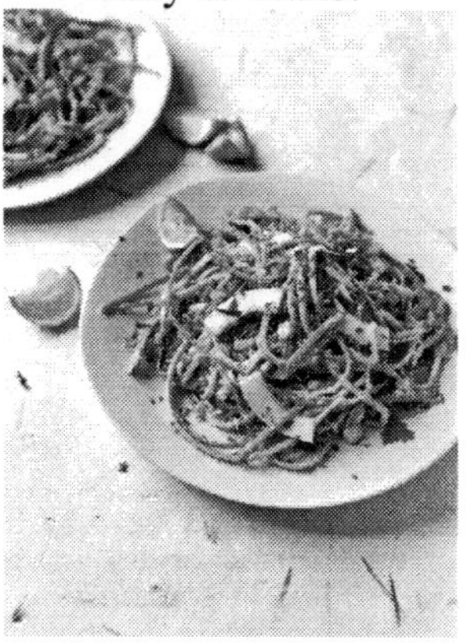

Ingredients:
2 green courgettes, cut into thin noodles
2 yellow courgettes, cut into thin noodles
2 carrots, cut into thin noodles
2 corn cobs
7 ounces of fresh peas
1sprig mixed coriander, rosemary, and parsley, finely chopped
For the coconut sauce:
1 shallot, chopped
Salt and black pepper
1 garlic clove, chopped
2 teaspoons of turmeric
Zest and juice from 1 lime
7 ounces of coconut milk
8 ounces of coconut water
4 ounces of desiccated coconut
1 teaspoon of curry powder
1 lime, cut into wedges

Directions:

1. In a bowl, mix shallot with ginger, garlic, turmeric, curry powder, coconut milk, coconut water, coconut, lime zest, and juice. Stir well.
2. Put everything in a food processor. Pulse a few times. Season with salt and pepper. Transfer into a bowl. Leave aside for now.
3. Place vegetable noodles in a bowl. Add corn and peas. Pour sauce over them. Sprinkle mixed herbs on top. Leave aside for 30 minutes. Transfer onto plates. Serve with lime wedges.

Enjoy!

Nutritional value: 598 calories, 36 grams of fat, 18 grams of protein, 53 grams of carbs, 16 grams of fiber

Asparagus and Special Mushroom Mayonnaise

This just can't get any better!

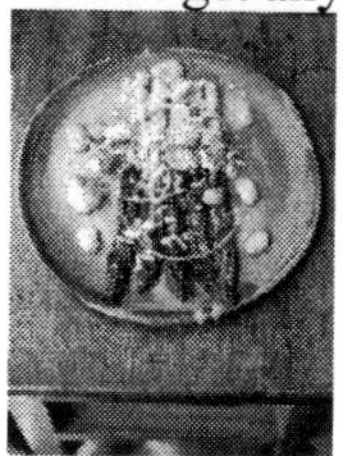

Ingredients:
16 asparagus spears
½ tablespoon of broad beans
1 tablespoon of cheddar cheese, crumbled
1 tablespoon of truffle oil
Salt and black pepper to taste
A sprigs watercress
For the mushroom mayonnaise:
7 ounces of button mushrooms
1 tablespoon of vegan mayonnaise
½ tablespoon of balsamic vinegar

Directions:

1. In a food processor, mix mushrooms with vinegar, and salt to taste. Pulse a few times.
2. Drain the excess liquid well. Transfer into a bowl. Mix with vegan mayo. Leave aside for now.
3. Place asparagus spears on heated grill. Cook for 3 minutes on one side and 2 on the other.
4. Divide beans on serving plates. Add asparagus and cheese. Drizzle some oil and the mushroom mayo on top.

Enjoy!

Nutritional value: 105 calories, 7 grams of fat, 2 grams of carbs, 2 grams of fiber, 6 grams of protein

Cauliflower Dhal

You'll fall in love with this vegetable!

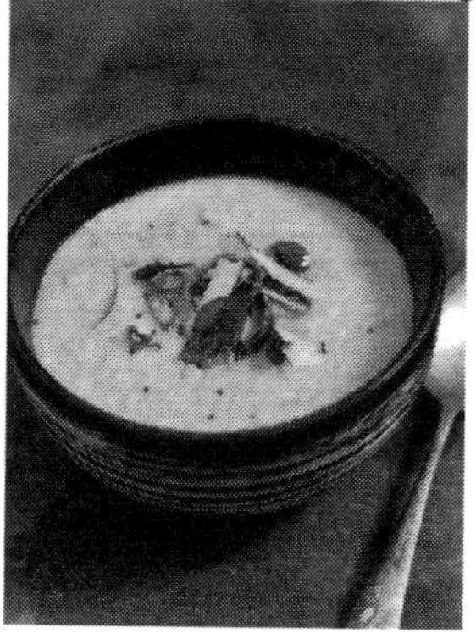

Ingredients:
4 shallots, chopped
1 garlic clove, chopped
1 cauliflower, cut into florets
A drizzle of groundnut oil
2 teaspoons of mustard seeds
1 sprigs curry leaves, chopped
8 ounces of yellow split peas
½ dried chili
28 ounces of canned coconut milk
Salt and pepper to taste

Directions:

1. Heat up a pan with a drizzle of oil, at a medium-high temperature. Add almost all shallots, almost all of the curry leaves, half of the mustard seeds, and the chili and garlic. Stir and cook for 3 minutes.
2. Add cauliflower, peas, coconut milk, some water, salt, and pepper. Stir. Bring to a boil. Reduce heat. Simmer for 40 minutes. Stir occasionally.
3. Heat up another pan with a drizzle of oil, at a medium-high temperature. Cook the rest of the shallots, curry leaves and mustard seeds for 3 minutes.
4. Transfer dhal into bowls. Serve with shallot mix on top.

Enjoy!

Nutritional value: 140 calories, 2 grams of fat, 20 grams of carbs, 4 grams of fiber, 9 grams of protein

Stir Fry Cabbage Mix

Simple and reenergizing

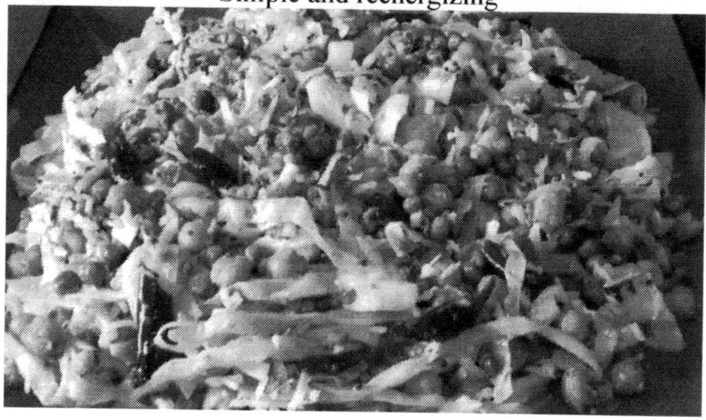

Ingredients:
3 tablespoons of extra-virgin olive oil
1 tablespoon of black lentils
2 dried red chilies, cut in pieces
1 teaspoon of Bengal garam
1 spring curry leaves, chopped
1 teaspoon of mustard seeds
1 pinch asafetida powder
1 cabbage head, finely chopped
4 green chili peppers, chopped
¼ cup of frozen peas
¼ coconut, grated
Salt and black pepper to taste

Directions:

1. Heat up a pan with the oil, at a medium-high temperature. Add red chili peppers, mustard seeds, black lentils, and Bengal gram. Stir. Fry for 3-4 minutes.
2. Add curry leaves, asafetida powder and green chili peppers. Stir. Cook for 1 more minute.
3. Add peas, cabbage, salt and black pepper. Stir. Fry for 10 minutes.
4. Add coconut. Cook for 2 more minutes. Transfer onto serving plates. Serve right away!

Enjoy!

Nutritional value: 232 calories, 4 grams of fat, 7 grams of carbs, 2 grams of fiber, 2 grams of protein

Chunky Vegetable Salad

A salad with large and juicy chunks of vegetables!

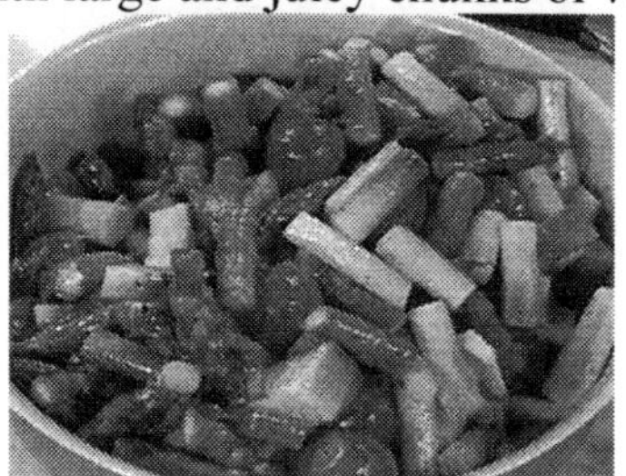

Ingredients:
1 small red onion, finely chopped
1 large red pepper, cut into chunks
½ pint grape tomatoes, cut in halves
1 medium cucumber, cut in chunks
2 celery ribs, cut into medium chunks
½ yellow squash, cut into medium chunks
3 tablespoons of extra-virgin olive oil
2 tablespoons of red wine vinegar
1 teaspoon of stevia
Salt and black pepper to taste
1 teaspoon of Italian seasoning

Directions:

1. In a bowl, mix tomatoes with bell pepper, red onion, celery, squash, and cucumber.
2. In a smaller bowl, mix olive oil with stevia, Italian seasoning, salt, pepper, and stevia. Stir well.
3. Mix salad with this dressing. Toss to coat. Serve right away!

Enjoy!

Nutritional value: 50 calories, 1 grams of fat, 6 grams of carbs, 1 grams of fiber, 2 grams of protein

Special Cauliflower and Chickpea Curry

A dish with a variety of textures and flavor!

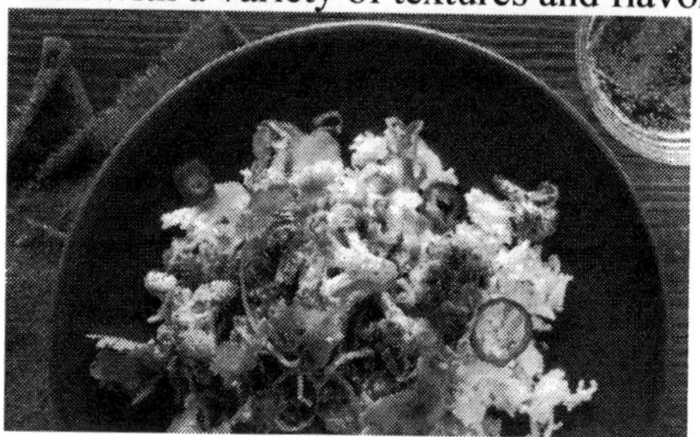

Ingredients:
2 Fresno chiles, thinly sliced
¼ teaspoon of coconut sugar
¼ cup of water
¼ cup of white vinegar
Salt and black pepper to taste
1 cauliflower, cut into small florets
¼ cup of extra-virgin olive oil
2 tablespoons of curry powder
2 shallots, finely sliced
¾ cup of vegetable oil
15 ounces of canned chickpeas, drained
1 yellow onion, chopped
A small piece of ginger, grated
2 teaspoons of tomato paste
1 teaspoon of lemongrass, grated
1 garlic clove, grated
1 teaspoon of harissa paste
13 ounces of canned coconut milk
¼ cup of water
1 tablespoon of fresh cilantro, chopped
Basmati rice for serving

Directions:

1. In a bowl, mix vinegar with chilies, sugar, salt, pepper and ¼ cup of water. Stir well. Leave aside for now.
2. In a baking dish, mix cauliflower with the olive oil, salt, and pepper. Put food in the oven at 450 degrees F. Bake for 35 minutes. Transfer onto paper towels. Drain fat. Put onto a plate. Leave aside.
3. Heat up a pan with ½ cup of vegetable oil, at a medium-high temperature. Cook shallots for 10 minutes. Stir occasionally. Transfer onto paper towels. Drain excess fat. Move food into a bowl. Season. Leave aside as well.
4. Heat up another pan with the rest of the vegetable oil, at a medium-high temperature. Cook onion for 5 minutes. Stir constantly.

5. Add garlic, ginger and lemongrass. Stir and cook for 1 more minute.
6. Add harissa paste and tomato paste. Stir and cook for 2 more minutes.
7. Add coconut milk. Bring to a boil. Cook until it thickens, for about 5 minutes.
8. Add chickpeas and ¼ cup of water. Stir. Bring to a boil again.
9. Remove mix from heat. Add cilantro and more salt and pepper. Stir.
10. Arrange basmati rice on serving plates. Add curry, roasted cauliflower, fried shallots, and chilies at the end.

Enjoy!

Nutritional value: 230 calories, 3 grams of fat, 10 grams of carbs, 4 grams of fiber, 13 grams of protein

Ricotta with Pomodoro Sauce

It's a unique recipe that tastes delicious!

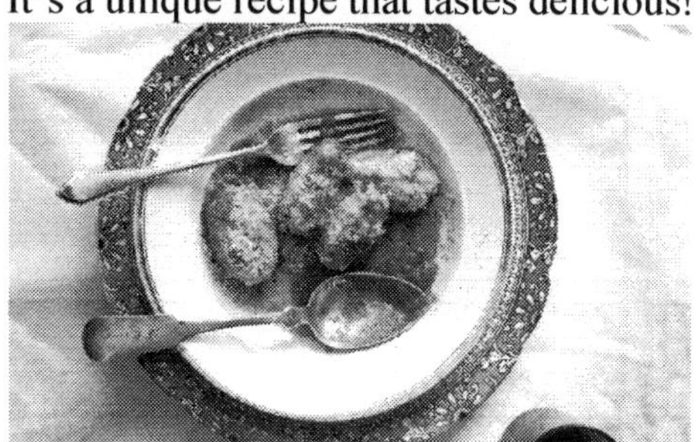

Ingredients:
2 cups of ricotta
1 egg, whisked
1 egg yolk, whisked
Salt and black pepper to taste
½ cup of parmesan, grated
½ cup of almond flour
For 3 cups of Pomodoro sauce:
28 ounces of canned tomatoes
½ cup of olive oil
2 garlic cloves, chopped
¼ teaspoon of stevia
A pinch of salt

Directions:

1. In your food processor, mix tomatoes with oil, garlic, stevia and a pinch of salt. Pulse a few times.
2. Transfer sauce into a pot. Bring to a boil. Cook for 2 minutes. Take off heat. Leave aside to cool down.
3. In a bowl, mix ricotta with egg yolk, egg, salt, pepper, and parmesan. Stir well.
4. Add ½ cup of almond flour. Stir well again.
5. Dust a working surface with some flour. Shape 30 balls from the dough you prepared earlier, using 2 spoons. Place them on the working surface. Then leave them aside for a few minutes.
6. Put some water in a pot. Bring to a boil. Add balls. Cook them for 6 minutes.
7. Divide them on serving plates. Add Pomodoro sauce on top. Serve.

Enjoy!

Nutritional value: calories 120, 4 grams of fat, 9 grams of carbs, 0 grams of fiber, 10 grams of protein

Chickpea Tagine and Figs

A vegetarian meal worth trying today!

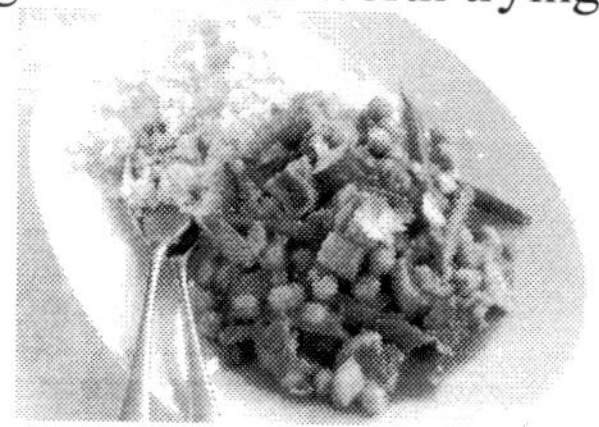

Ingredients:
1 yellow onion, finely chopped
2 tablespoons of extra-virgin olive oil
2 garlic cloves, finely chopped
2 teaspoons of spice mix
28 ounces of canned chickpeas, drained
14 ounces of canned tomatoes, chopped
2 cups of vegetable stock
2 zucchinis finely, chopped
6 ounces of green beans, cut in halves
2 cups of couscous, already cooked
2 tablespoons of coriander, finely chopped
½ cup of figs, dried and chopped
Salt and pepper to taste

Directions:

1. Heat up a pan with the oil, at a medium-high temperature. Cook the onion for 3-4 minutes.
2. Add garlic, spice mix, salt and pepper. Stir and cook for 5 minutes.
3. Add tomato, stock and chickpeas. Bring to a boil. Cover. Reduce heat. Simmer for 10 minutes.
4. Add beans, figs and zucchinis. Stir and cook for 8 more minutes.
5. Divide couscous on serving plates. Add vegetable mix Top with chopped coriander.

Enjoy!

Nutritional value: 300 calories, 15 grams of fat, 20 grams of carbs, 19 grams of fiber, 24 grams of protein

Caramelized Onion Tart

A hearty and healthy recipe!

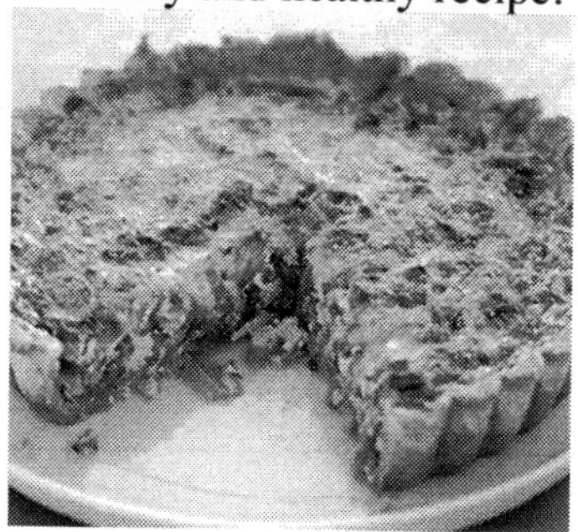

Ingredients:
14 ounces of vegetarian puff pastry
¼ cup of Country Crock Original
2 yellow onion, thinly sliced
Salt and black pepper to taste
2 tablespoons of Stevia
10 thyme sprigs, chopped
8 ounces of goat cheese, crumbled

Directions:

1. Roll puff pastry on a floured working surface. Transfer it onto a lined baking sheet. Prick with a fork. Put food in the oven at 400 degrees F. Bake for 15 minutes. Take out of the oven. Leave aside to cool down.
2. Put Country Crock Original in a pot. Warm it up at a medium-high temperature. Add onion. Cook for 10 minutes.
3. Add stevia, salt, and black pepper. Stir and cook for 5 more minutes.
4. Take onion mix off heat. Spread over pastry. Sprinkle goat cheese and thyme on top. Put food in the oven again. Bake for 10 minutes.
5. Take out of the oven. Leave aside to cool down. Cut and serve

Enjoy!

Nutritional value: 160 calories, 2 grams of fat. 18 grams of carbs, 1 grams of fiber, 2 grams of protein

Special Vegetable Pies

Don't skip dinner! Try this wonderful pie!

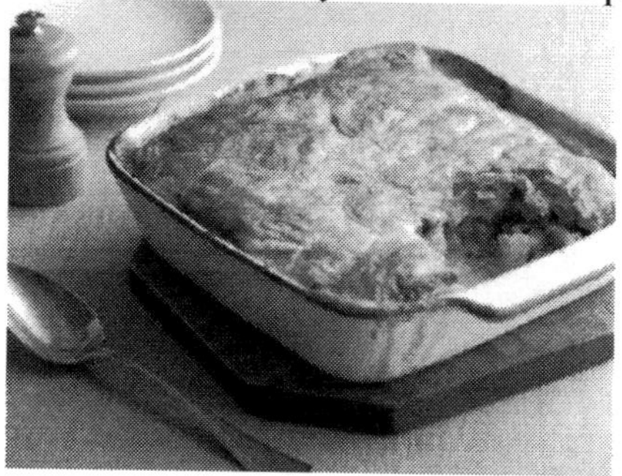

Ingredients:
4 potatoes, chopped
¾ cup of unsalted butter
Salt and black pepper to taste
1 leek, sliced
1 yellow onion, chopped
1 fennel bulb, chopped
¾ cup of almond flour
3 and ½ cups of vegetable broth
1 tablespoon of thyme, finely chopped
1 tablespoon of oregano, finely chopped
¼ cup of parsley, finely chopped
4 ounces of white mushrooms, sliced
5 carrots, chopped
¼ cup of coconut milk
1½ cup of frozen peas
1 egg mixed with 1 tablespoon of water

Directions;

1. Put potatoes in a pan. Cover with water. Add salt. Place food on the stove. Heat up at a medium-high temperature. Bring to a boil. Cook for 8 minutes. Drain. Leave aside.
2. Add vegan butter to a large pot. Melt. Add onion, leek, fennel, salt, and pepper. Stir and cook for 8 minutes. Add flour. Cook for 4 more minutes.
3. Add vegetable broth, thyme, parsley, oregano, peas, mushrooms, carrots, potatoes, salt, and pepper. Stir and cook for 10 minutes. Add coconut milk. Stir and cook for 15 more minutes.
4. Roll out puff pastry on a floured working surface. Cut 8 circles. Fill 8 ramekins with the vegetable mix you prepared earlier. Top with pastry circles. Seal edges. Brush each with egg mixed with water. Sprinkle salt and pepper. Put food in the oven at 400 degrees F. Bake for 25 minutes.
5. Take them out of the oven. Leave aside for 5 minutes. Serve!

Enjoy!

Nutritional value: 420 calories, 19 grams of fat, 54 grams of carbs, 4 grams of fiber, 9 grams of protein

Vegetarian Maple Cupcakes

They're so delicious! We just love them!

Ingredients:
4 tablespoons of coconut butter
4 eggs
½ cup of applesauce
2 teaspoons of cinnamon
1 teaspoon of vanilla extract
½ an apple, sliced
4 teaspoons of maple syrup
¾ cup of almond flour
½ teaspoon of baking powder
Cinnamon for serving
A pinch of salt

Directions:

1. Heat up a pan with the butter, at a medium temperature. Add applesauce, vanilla, eggs and maple syrup. Stir. Take off heat. Leave aside to cool down.
2. When it's cold enough, add almond flour, cinnamon, baking powder and a pinch of salt. Stir. Pour into a cupcake pan lined with parchment paper. Put food in the oven at 350 degrees F. Bake for 20 minutes.
3. Take out of the oven. Leave them to cool. Transfer to a platter. Top with apple slices and cinnamon. Serve!

Enjoy!

Nutritional value: 150 calories, 3 grams of fat, 5 grams of carbs, 0 grams of fiber, 4 grams of protein

Baked Apples

The perfect dessert!

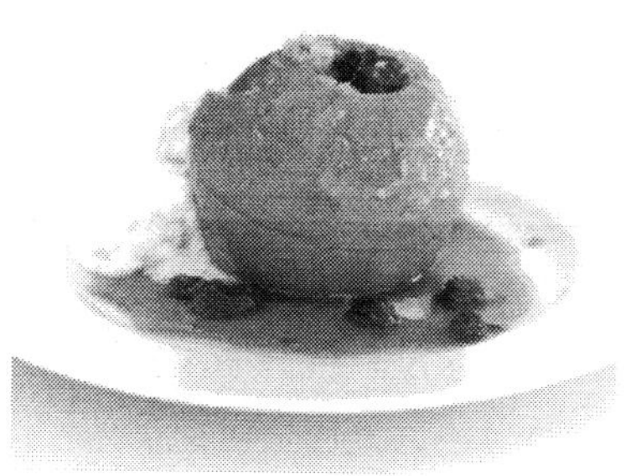

Ingredients:
4 apples cored
Honey to taste
1 tablespoon of cinnamon

Directions:

1. Fill apples with raisins. Top with cinnamon. Drizzle some honey on them.
2. Put them in an ovenproof dish. Bake them in the oven at 375 degrees F for 20 minutes.
3. Take them out of the oven. Cool apples for 3-4 minutes. Serve.

Enjoy!

Nutritional value: 127 calories, 4 grams of fat, 25 grams of carbs, 2 grams of fiber, 1 grams of protein

Pumpkin Cookies

A special dessert for a special occasion!

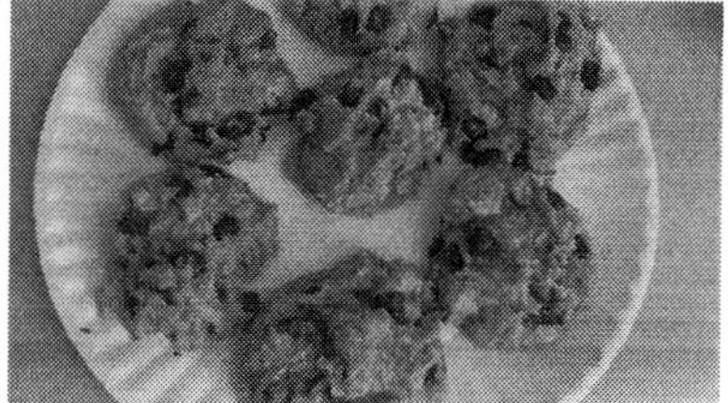

Ingredients:
2 and ½ cups of almond flour
½ teaspoon of baking soda
½ cup of pumpkin flesh, already mashed
A pinch of salt
3 tablespoons of cold water
2 tablespoons of coconut butter
1 tablespoon of ground flax seeds
1 teaspoon of vanilla extract
¼ cup of honey
½ cup of vegetarian chocolate chips

Directions:

1. Mix flax seeds with cold water in a bowl. Leave aside for now.
2. In another bowl, mix flour with salt and baking soda. Leave aside.
3. In a different bowl, combine honey with pumpkin mash, vanilla, butter, and flax seeds. Stir.
4. Mix flour with pumpkin mash and chocolate chips. Stir well.
5. Put 1 tablespoon of cookie dough on a baking dish and flatten it.
6. Repeat this with the rest of the dough. Put food in the oven at 350 degrees F. Bake for 15 minutes. Take out of the oven. Leave aside for a few minutes. Transfer to a platter. Serve!

Enjoy!

Nutritional value: 131 calories, 4 grams of fat, 22 grams of carbs, 0 grams of fiber, 1 grams of protein

Tasty Curd

So fresh and delicious!

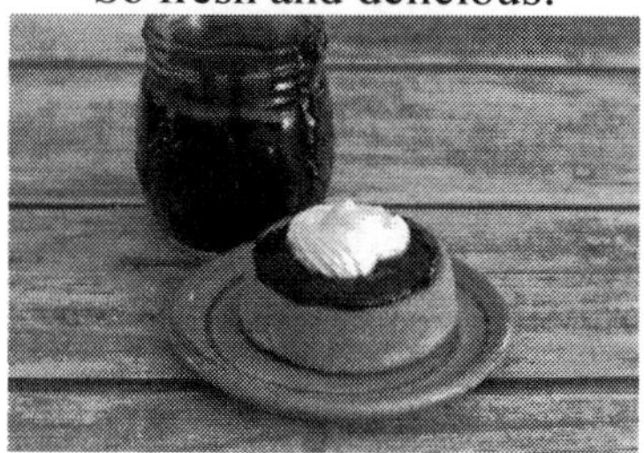

Ingredients:
2 cups of blueberries
2/3 cup of Stevia
¼ cup of lemon juice
4 tablespoons of coconut butter
2 teaspoons of lemon zest
3 egg yolks

Directions:

1. Heat up blueberries and lemon juice in a pan at a medium-high temperature. Stir. Bring to a boil. Cook for 3-4 minutes.
2. Transfer into a strainer. Place into a bowl and mash, then place into a double broiler. Add some water. Bring to a simmer. Boil for 4-5 minutes more.
3. Add sugar and butter and mix well.
4. Whisk eggs and add them to blueberry mix.
5. Stir curd. Heat up at 175 degrees F. Keep for 2-3 minutes.
6. Pour into small cups. Leave to cool down. Serve!

Enjoy!

Nutritional value: 80 calories, 0 grams of fat, 9 grams of carbs, 0 grams of fiber, 0 grams of protein

Delicious Rhubarb Pie

It's a fabulous dessert!

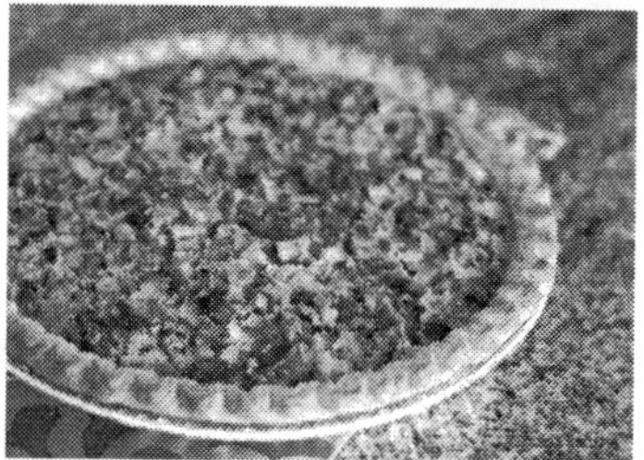

Ingredients:
1 and ¼ cups of almond flour
8 tablespoons of coconut butter
A pinch of salt
5 tablespoons of cold water
1 teaspoon of palm sugar
For the filling:
3 cups of rhubarb, finely chopped
3 tablespoons of almond flour
1½ cups of palm sugar
2 eggs
A pinch of salt
½ teaspoon of nutmeg
1 tablespoon of coconut butter
2 tablespoons of almond milk

Directions:

1. Mix 1 and ¼ cups of flour with salt and 1 teaspoon of sugar in a bowl.
2. Add 8 tablespoons of butter and the cold water. Stir until you obtain a dough.
3. Transfer dough onto a floured working surface. Shape a disk. Flatten. Wrap in plastic. Keep in the fridge for about 30 minutes.
4. Take out the dough and roll it. Transfer onto a pie plate. Leave aside for a few minutes.
5. In a bowl, mix rhubarb with a pinch of salt, 1½ cups of sugar, nutmeg and 3 tablespoons of flour. Stir.
6. In a second bowl, whisk eggs with milk.
7. Add this to rhubarb mix. Stir well. Pour into pie shell. Bake in the oven for 50 minutes at 400 degrees F.
8. Take out of the oven. Leave it to cool down, then cut and serve it.

Enjoy!

Nutritional value: 300 calories, 20 grams of fat, 20 grams of carbs, 2 grams of fiber, 3 grams of protein

Cherry Cobbler

It's a delightful dessert!

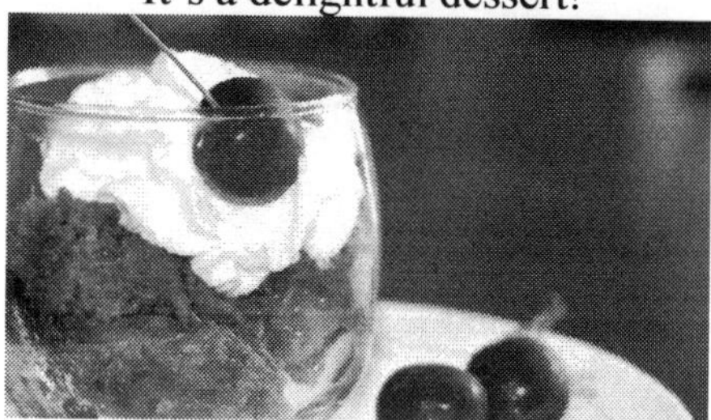

Ingredients:
1 cup of almond flour
½ cup of coconut butter
1 cup of palm sugar
2 cups of cherries, already pitted
1 teaspoon of baking powder
¾ cup of Stevia
1 cup of almond milk
1 tablespoon of almond flour

Directions:

1. Place coconut butter in an oven-proof dish. Put food in the oven at 350 degrees for 5 minutes. Take it out. Leave aside for now.
2. In a bowl, mix 1 cup of almond flour with 1 cup of palm sugar, baking powder, and milk. Stir well. Pour over butter. Leave aside.
3. Place cherries in a bowl. Mix with 1 tablespoon of almond flour and stevia. Toss to coat. Pour evenly over batter in the baking dish. Put food in the oven at 350 degrees F. Bake for 1 hour.
4. Take out of the oven. Cool cobbler. Cut. Transfer to a platter. Serve!

Enjoy!

Nutritional value: 235 calories, 2 grams of fat, 30 grams of carbs, 2 grams of fiber, 5 grams of protein

Fruit Salad

A simple 100% vegetarian recipe!

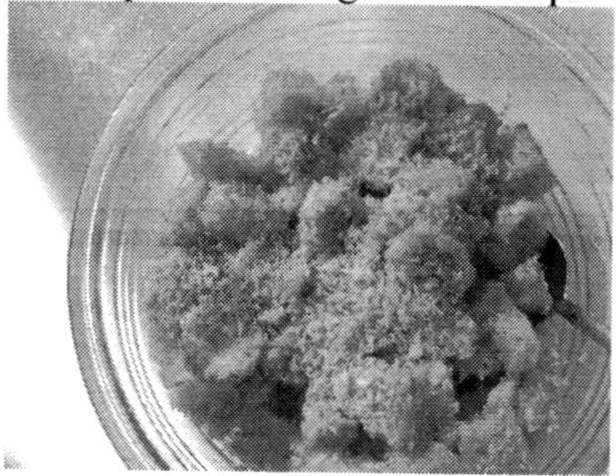

Ingredients:
2 cups of pineapple, chopped
1 cup of mango, diced
1 cup of orange, sliced
1 cup of banana, sliced
1 tablespoon of palm sugar
1 tablespoon of lime juice
1/8 teaspoon of cinnamon
1/8 teaspoon of ginger, grated
1/8 teaspoon of cardamom
1 cup of coconut, toasted for serving

Directions:

1. In a bowl, mix pineapple with banana, mango, and orange.
2. Add sugar, lime juice, cinnamon, ginger and cardamom. Toss to coat.
3. Sprinkle grated coconut on top. Keep in the fridge until you serve!

Enjoy!

Nutritional value: 270 calories, 14 grams of fat, 38 grams of carbs, 7 grams of fiber, 3 grams of protein

Fruit Jelly

Who wouldn't like this?

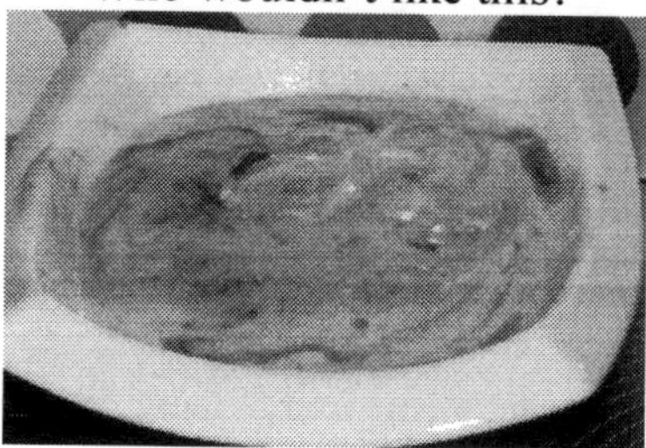

Ingredients:
1/3 pound red fruit jelly
1/5 pound coconut yogurt.
A sprigs fresh berries
A sprigs nut pieces

Directions:

1. In your food processor, mix fruit jelly with yogurt. Pulse a few times.
2. Add berries and nuts. Toss to coat. Serve right away!

Enjoy!

Nutritional value: 70 calories, 29 grams of fat, 4 grams of carbs, 0 grams of fiber, 3 grams of protein

Couscous Dessert

It's an Egyptian style dessert you just have to try!

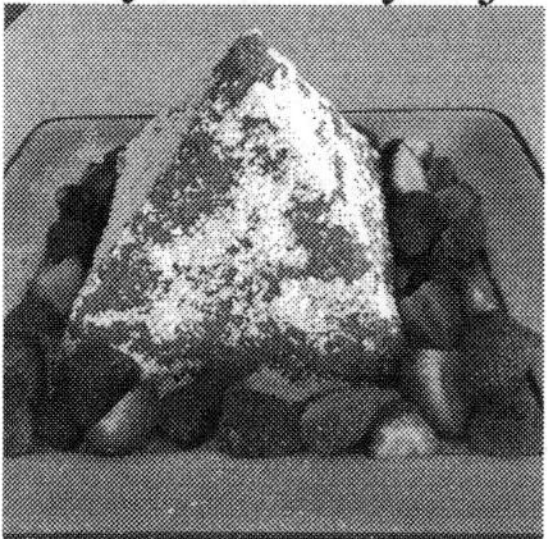

Ingredients:
1 cup of couscous
2 tablespoons of rose water
2 cups of fruit juice
3 tablespoons of coconut butter
¼ cup of pistachio, grated
¼ cup of almonds, blanched
½ cup of palm sugar
1 tablespoon of cinnamon
½ cup of pomegranate seeds

Directions:

1. In a pot, mix fruit juice with rose water and couscous. Bring to a boil. Cover. Take off heat. Leave aside for 15 minutes. Fluff with a fork.
2. Add melted coconut butter. Stir well.
3. Also, add almonds and pistachios. Stir.
4. Transfer onto plates. Sprinkle palm sugar, cinnamon, and pomegranate seeds.

Enjoy!

Nutritional value: 276 calories, 11 grams of fat, 38 grams of carbs, 3 grams of fiber, 6 grams of protein

Fruit Cocktail

Are you in the mood for a tasty cocktail? Try a fruit cocktail!

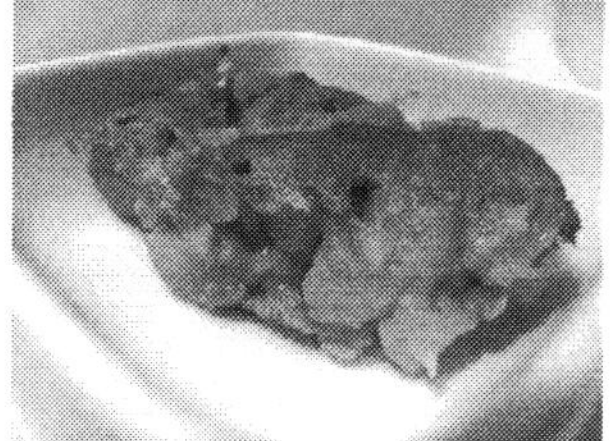

Ingredients:
16 ounces of canned fruit mix, drained and juice reserved
9 ounces of vegetarian yellow cake mix
Cooking spray

Directions:

1. In a bowl, mix fruit juice with cake mix. Stir well.
2. Add fruit mix. Toss to coat. Pour into a baking pan sprayed with some oil.
3. Put food in the oven at 350 degrees F. Bake for 45 minutes.
4. Take out of the oven. Leave aside to cool down. Then serve!

Enjoy!

Nutritional value: 320 calories, 7 grams of fat, 60 grams of carbs, 1 grams of fiber, 3 grams of protein

Fig and Almond Dessert

Simple, tasty, vegetarian

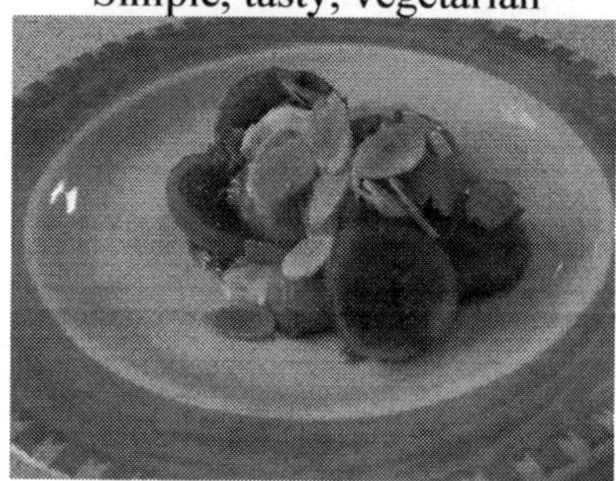

Ingredients:
2 tablespoons of coconut butter
12 figs, cut in halves
¼ cup of palm sugar
1 cup of almonds, blanched and toasted

Directions:
1. Put butter in a pot over high heat. Melt it.
2. Add figs and sugar. Stir. Cook for 4 minutes.
3. Add almonds. Toss to coat. Transfer into bowls. Serve!

Enjoy!

Nutritional value: 420 calories, 25 grams of fat, 49 grams of carbs, 7 grams of fiber, 9 grams of protein

Avocado Dessert Salad

Are you willing to try a different dessert this time?

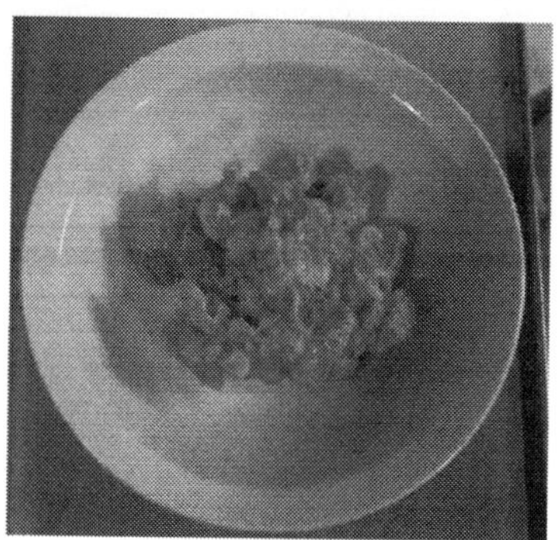

Ingredients:
4 bananas, chopped
5 avocados, chopped
Juice from 2 lemons
4 tablespoons of palm sugar

Directions:

1. Put avocados and bananas in a bowl. Mash with a fork.
2. Add lemon juice and palm sugar. Toss to coat.
3. Taste. Add more sugar and lemon juice if needed.
4. Keep in the fridge until you serve!

Enjoy!

Nutritional value: 300 calories, 21 grams of fat, 34 grams of carbs, 12 grams of fiber, 3 grams of protein

Vegetarian Sponge Cake

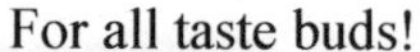
For all taste buds!

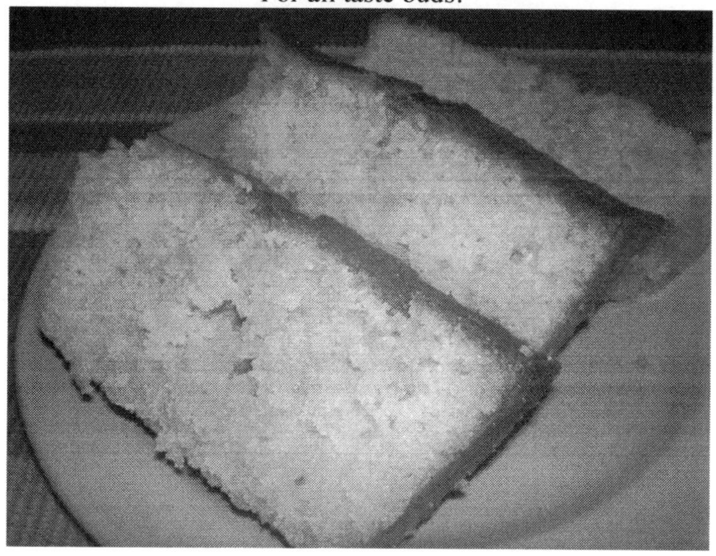

Ingredients:
3 cups of almond flour
3 teaspoons of baking powder
½ cup of cornstarch
1 teaspoon of baking soda
1 cup of vegetable oil
1½ cup of soy milk
1 2/3 cup of palm sugar
2 cups of water
¼ cup of lemon juice
2 teaspoons of vanilla extract

Directions:

1. In a bowl, mix flour with cornstarch, baking powder, baking soda, and sugar. Stir well.
2. In another bowl, mix oil with soy milk, water, vanilla, and lemon juice. Stir.
3. Combine the two mixtures. Whisk together. Pour into a sprayed baking dish. Put food in the oven at 357 degrees F. Bake for 20 minutes.
4. Take out of the oven. Leave the cake to cool down. Cut and serve!

Enjoy!

Nutritional value: 346 calories, 16 grams of fat, 47 grams of carbs, 0 grams of fiber, 2 grams of protein

Pumpkin Pie

Sometimes, a pumpkin pie is all you need!

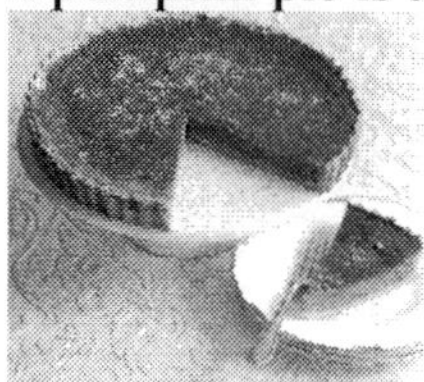

Ingredients:
2 boxes silken tofu
2 cup of already cooked pumpkin flesh
1½ cup of palm sugar
A pinch of salt
2 vegan pie crusts
For the pumpkin spice:
1 teaspoon of ginger, grated
2 teaspoons of cinnamon
1 teaspoon of ground cloves
1 teaspoon of allspice
2 teaspoons of nutmeg

Directions:

1. Mix tofu in your food processor until it's smooth (~ 4 minutes).
2. Add pumpkin flesh. Pulse again well.
3. Transfer paste into a bowl. Mix with sugar, cinnamon, ginger, cloves, nutmeg, allspice and a pinch of salt. Stir well.
4. Pour this into pie crusts. Put food in the oven at 375 degrees F. Bake for 45 minutes.
5. Take out of the oven. Leave aside to cool down. Cut and serve!

Enjoy!

Nutritional value: 375 calories, 11 grams of fat, 45 grams of carbs, 2 grams of fiber, 5 grams of protein

Apple and Pumpkin Dessert

Apple and pumpkin is an extremely delicious combination!

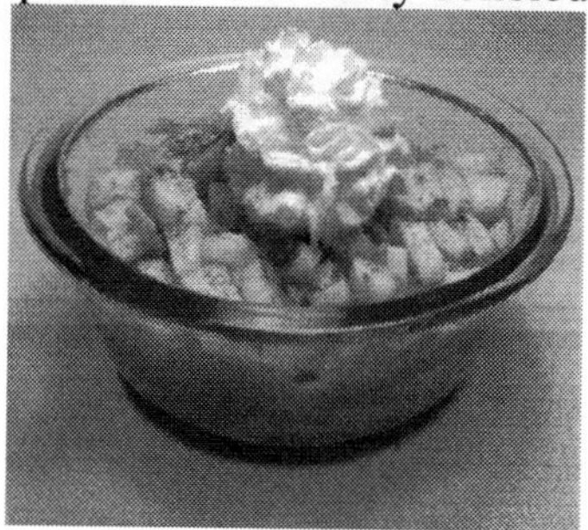

Ingredients:
1 apple, chopped
¼ cup of canned pumpkin flesh
2 tablespoons of water
A pinch of pumpkin spice

Directions:

1. In a bowl, mix some apple slices with some of the pumpkin flesh.
2. Sprinkle pumpkin spice. Layer the rest of the apples and the pumpkin. Top with pumpkin spice again.
3. Add water. Put food in the microwave. Put the heat on and wait 4 minutes.
4. Serve right away!

Enjoy!

Nutritional value: 99 calories, 0 grams of fat, 25 grams of carbs, 5 grams of fiber, 1 gram of protein

Blueberry and Coconut Cake

For when you are craving something sweet and satisfying!

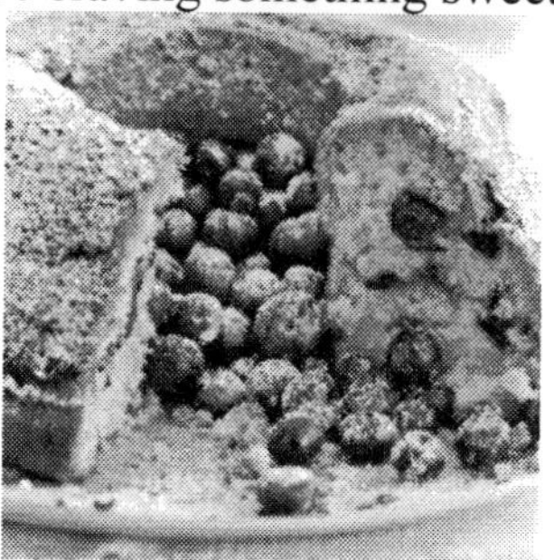

Ingredients:
3 eggs
2 teaspoons of vanilla sugar
8 ounces of rice bran oil
7 ounces of palm sugar
1½ cups of almond flour
1 cup of soy milk
1½ tablespoon of desiccated coconut
½ cup of fresh blueberries, and some more for serving

Directions:

1. In a bowl, mix oil with sugar, vanilla, and eggs. Stir well.
2. In another bowl, mix coconut with flour.
3. Add this to the oil and sugar mix.
4. Also, add soy milk. Stir well.
5. Spoon half of the batter into a pan. Add blueberries. Stir gently. Add the rest of the batter. Put food in the oven at 357 degrees F. Bake for 1 hour.
6. Take out of the oven. Leave aside to cool down. Cut and serve!

Enjoy!

Nutritional value: 387 calories, 24 grams of fat, 47 grams of carbs, 2 grams of fiber, 5 grams of protein

Baked Nectarine and Almond Dessert

It's an easy to make dessert!

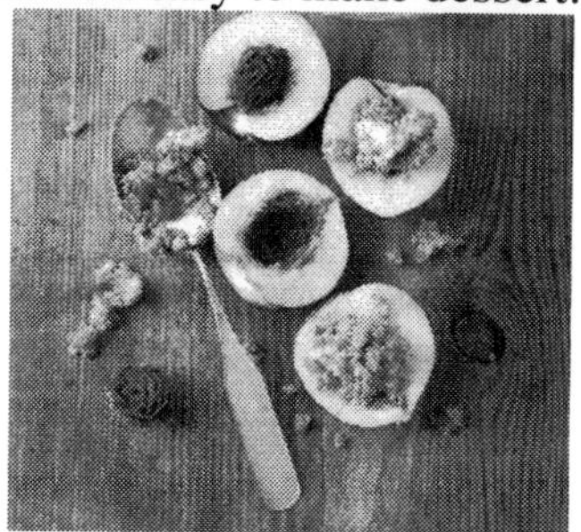

Ingredients:
6 nectarines cut in halves
3 ounces of amaretti biscuits
3 ounces of coconut butter, softened
2 and ½ ounces of almonds
2 and ½ ounces of palm sugar
2 tablespoons of toasted almonds
1 egg
1 cup of marsala
Coconut yogurt for serving

Directions:

1. Put nectarine halves in a baking dish. Leave aside.
2. In a bowl, crumb amaretti biscuits and mix them with butter, almonds, sugar and egg. Stir well.
3. Put some of this mixture in each nectarine half. Sprinkle toasted almonds. Pour marsala on top. Put food in the oven at 350 degrees F. Bake for 40 minutes.
4. Take out of the oven. Leave nectarines to cool down. Top with coconut yogurt. Serve!

Enjoy!

Nutritional value: 447 calories, 25 grams of fat, 45 grams of carbs, 3 grams of fiber, 7 grams of protein

Vegetarian Passion Fruit Pudding

If you love pudding you will love this recipe!

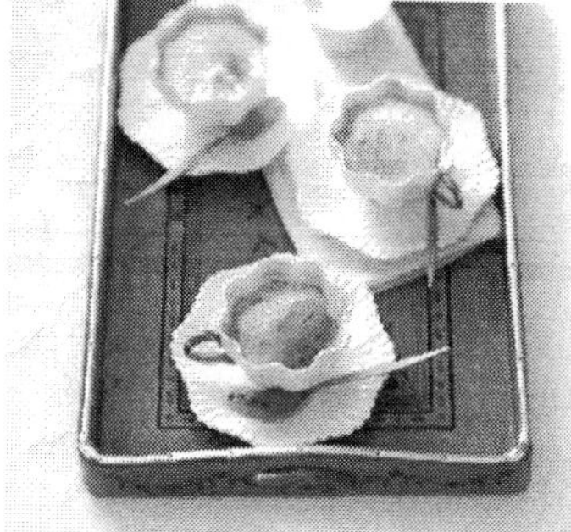

Ingredients:
1 cup of passion fruit curds
4 passion fruits, pulp, and seeds
3 and ½ ounces of palm sugar
3 eggs
2 ounces of melted butter
3 and ½ ounces of soy milk
½ cup of almond flour
½ teaspoon of baking powder

Directions:

1. Put half of the passionfruit curd in a bowl. Leave aside.
2. In another bowl, mix the rest of the curd with passionfruit seeds. Pulp. Stir.
3. Divide this into 6 teacups.
4. In a bowl, whisk eggs with sugar, butter, the reserved curd, baking powder, milk, and flour. Stir well.
5. Divide this into 6 cups. Put them in an oven pan. Fill the pan halfway with water. Put food in the oven at 200 degrees F. Bake for 50 minutes.
6. Take puddings out of the oven. Leave aside to cool down. Serve!

Enjoy!

Nutritional value: 430 calories, 22 grams of fat, 52 grams of carbs, 2 grams of fiber, 8 grams of protein

Cornbread Muffins

This is a brilliant dessert recipe!

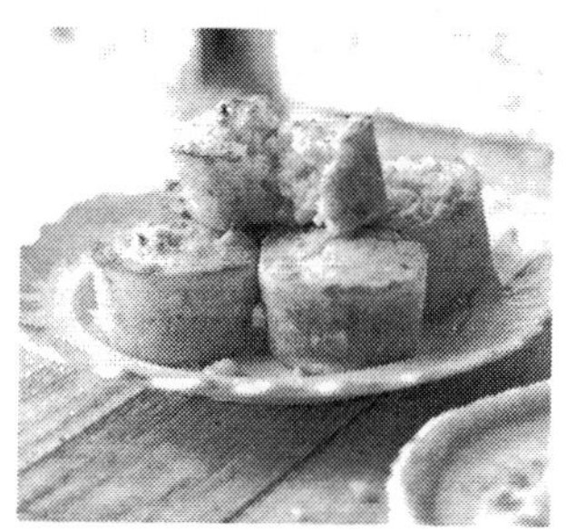

Ingredients:
3 cup of almond flour
1 cup of cornmeal
1 cup of palm sugar
2 tablespoons of baking powder
A pinch of salt
1½ cups of soy milk
½ pound coconut butter
2 eggs

Directions:

1. In a bowl, mix flour with cornmeal, sugar, salt, and baking powder.
2. In another bowl, mix butter with milk and eggs.
3. Combine the two mixtures. Stir well.
4. Spoon batter into 12 muffin cups lined with parchment paper.
5. Put food them in the oven at 350 degrees F. Bake for 30 minutes.
6. Take them out of the oven. Leave aside to cool down. Transfer to a platter. Serve!

Enjoy!

Nutritional value: 345 calories, 9 grams of fat, 57 grams of carbs, 3 grams of fiber, 6 grams of protein

Fruits with Orange Vinaigrette

A healthy option for dessert!

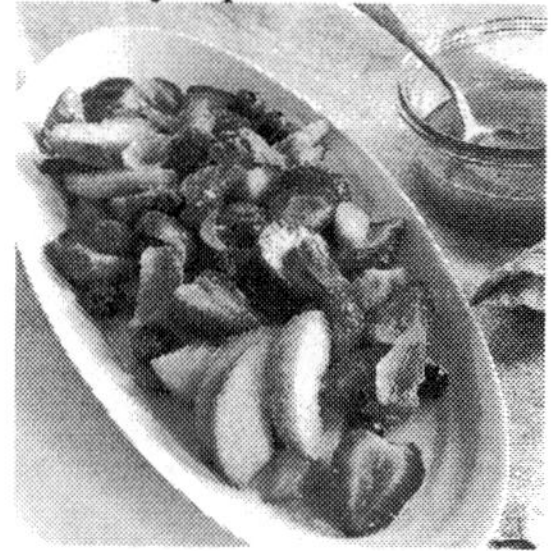

Ingredients:
1 cup of orange juice
1½ tablespoons of palm sugar
1½ tablespoons of champagne vinegar
A pinch of salt
1 tablespoon of olive oil
1 pound of strawberries, cut in halves
1½ cups of blueberries
1 peach, cut into 16 wedges
¼ cup of basil leaves

Directions:

1. In a pot, mix orange juice with sugar and vinegar. Bring to a boil over a medium-high temperature. Simmer for 15 minutes. Add oil and a pinch of salt. Stir. Leave aside for 2 minutes.
2. In a bowl, mix blueberries with strawberries and peach wedges. Add orange vinaigrettes. Toss to coat. Sprinkle basil on top. Serve!

Enjoy!

Nutritional value: 163 calories, 4 grams of fat, 32 grams of carbs, 4 grams of fiber, 2 grams of protein

Delicious Cherry Sorbet

It's a unique tasting sorbet!

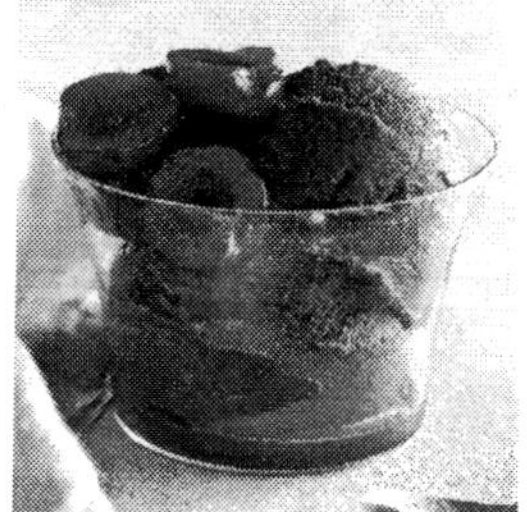

Ingredients:
½ cup of vegetarian cocoa
¾ cup of red cherry jam
¼ cup of palm sugar
2 cups of water
A pinch of salt
For the compote:
¼ cup of palm sugar
1 pound of cherries pitted, cut in halves

Directions:

1. In a pan, mix cherry jam with cocoa, sugar and a pinch of salt. Stir. Bring to a boil. Gradually add the water. Stir again. Remove from heat. Leave aside to cool down completely.
2. Whisk this sorbet again. Pour into a casserole. Keep in the freezer for 1 hour.
3. For the compote, mix in a bowl, ¼ cup of palm sugar with cherries. Toss to coat. Leave aside for 1 hour.
4. When the time has passed, serve this compote with the sorbet.

Enjoy!

Nutritional value: 197 calories, 1 grams of fat, 50 grams of carbs, 3 grams of fiber, 1 grams of protein

Vegetarian Apricot Sorbet

Cool and refreshing!

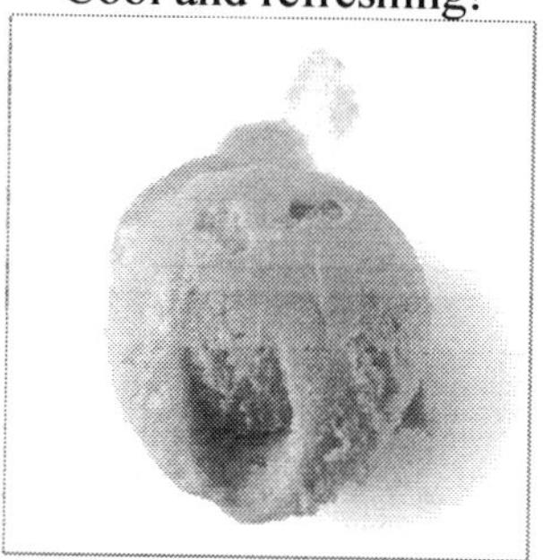

Ingredients:
2 cups of sparkling wine
1 cup of palm sugar
2 strips lemon peel
A pinch of salt
1½ pounds apricots pitted, cut in halves

Directions:

1. Heat up a saucepan at a medium-high temperature. Add sugar, wine, apricots, lemon peel and a pinch of salt.
2. Stir. Bring to a boil. Simmer for 10 minutes. Remove from heat. Discard lemon peel. Leave aside to cool down.
3. Transfer mix into a food processor. Pulse very well.
4. Put this in a casserole. Put food in the freezer. Leave there for 2 hours.
5. Take out of the freezer and serve!

Enjoy!

Nutritional value: 178 calories, 0 grams of fat, sodium 19

Mango Granita

It's a tropical vegetarian dessert!

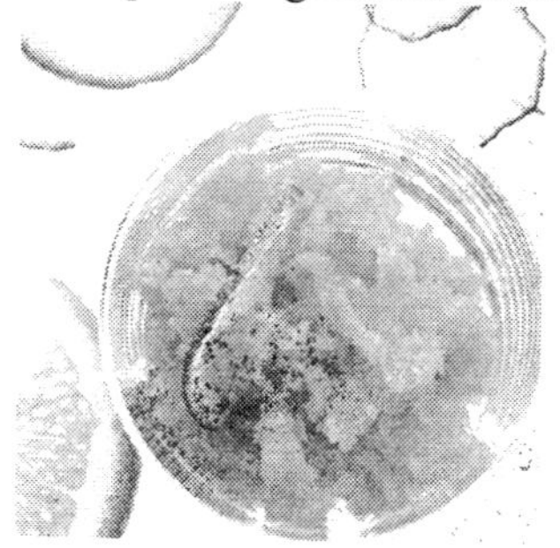

Ingredients:
4 cups of mango, peeled and cubed
¼ cup of orange juice
6 tablespoons of palm sugar
3 tablespoons of lime juice
A pinch of salt
A pinch of ground red pepper

Directions:

1. Put mango, orange and lime juice, sugar, salt and red pepper in a pan. Bring to a boil. Stir. Reduce heat to low. Simmer for 10 minutes.
2. Remove from heat. Leave aside for 10 minutes. Pour into your food processor. Pulse a few times. Strain into a bowl. Discard solids. Pour mix into a baking dish. Put food in the freezer and keep it there for 6 hours. Scrape once every hour.
3. Scrape with a fork after 6 hours. Serve!

Enjoy!

Nutritional value: 127 calories, 0 grams of fat, 33 grams of carbs, 2 grams of fiber, 0 grams of protein

Apple Crisp

Super nutritious!

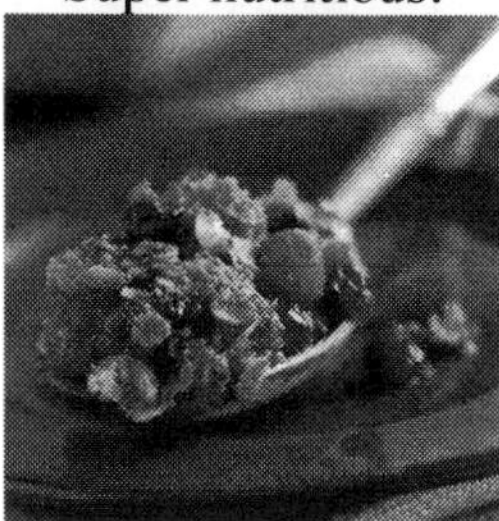

Ingredients:
2 cup of cranberries
3 cups of apples, cubed
Cooking spray
½ cup of palm sugar
1/3 cup of almond flour
1 cup of oats
¼ canola oil
½ cup of palm sugar

Directions:

1. In a bowl, mix apple cubes with cranberries and ½ cup of sugar. Stir well.
2. Spray a baking dish with oil. Leave aside.
3. In another bowl, mix flour with oats, canola oil and ½ cup of sugar. Stir well.
4. Pour apple mix into the baking dish. Sprinkle flour mix on top. Put food in the oven at 350 degrees F. Bake for 40 minutes.
5. Take apple crisp out of the oven. Leave aside to cool down. Serve!

Enjoy!

Nutritional value: 202 calories, 6 grams of fat, 36 grams of carbs, 3 grams of fiber, 2 grams of protein

Grapefruit Granita

Everyone will love this recipe!

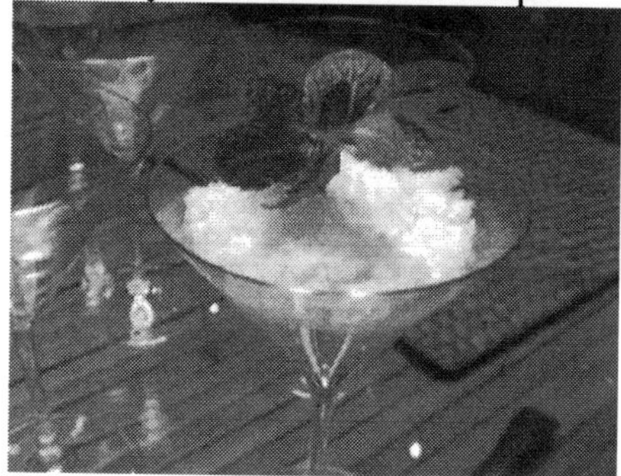

Ingredients:
1 cup of water
1 cup of palm sugar
½ cup of mint, chopped
64 ounces of red grapefruit juice
Mint leaves for serving

Directions:

1. Put 1 cup of water in a pan. Bring to a boil. Add sugar. Stir. Take off heat.
2. Add mint. Cover. Leave aside for 5 minutes.
3. Strain into a plastic container. Discard mint. Add grapefruit juice. Cover. Put food in the freezer for 4 hours.
4. Take out of the freezer 15 minutes before you scrape with a fork. Serve with mint leaves on top.
5. Enjoy!

Nutritional value: 120, 0 grams of fat, 2 grams of carbs, 0 grams of fiber, 1 grams of protein

Made in the USA
Middletown, DE
17 March 2017